2013

Fam Violence

What Health Care Providers Need to Know

Rose S. Fife, MD, MPH

Barbara F. Kampen Professor of Women's Health
Professor of Medicine and Biochemistry
and Molecular Biology
School of Medicine
Indiana University
Co-Director, IU Family Violence Institute

Sarina Schrager, MD, MS

Associate Professor (CHS)
School of Medicine and Public Health
University of Wisconsin

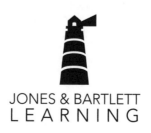

JONES & BARTLETT
L E A R N I N G

World Headquarters

Jones & Bartlett Learning	Jones & Bartlett Learning	Jones & Bartlett Learning
40 Tall Pine Drive	Canada	International
Sudbury, MA 01776	6339 Ormindale Way	Barb House, Barb Mews
978-443-5000	Mississauga, Ontario L5V 1J2	London W6 7PA
info@jblearning.com	Canada	United Kingdom
www.jblearning.com		

Jones & Bartlett Learning books and products are available through most bookstores and online booksellers. To contact Jones & Bartlett Learning directly, call 800-832-0034, fax 978-443-8000, or visit our website, www.jblearning.com.

Substantial discounts on bulk quantities of Jones & Bartlett Learning publications are available to corporations, professional associations, and other qualified organizations. For details and specific discount information, contact the special sales department at Jones & Bartlett Learning via the above contact information or send an email to specialsales@jblearning.com.

This publication is designed to provide accurate and authoritative information in regard to the Subject Matter covered. It is sold with the understanding that the publisher is not engaged in rendering legal, accounting, or other professional service. If legal advice or other expert assistance is required, the service of a competent professional person should be sought.

Production Credits
Publisher: David Cella
Associate Editor: Maro Gartside
Production Director: Amy Rose
Senior Production Editor: Renée Sekerak
Marketing Manager: Grace Richards
Manufacturing and Inventory Control Supervisor: Amy Bacus
Composition: Glyph International
Cover Design: Kate Ternullo
Cover Images: Banner of hands © Christopher Jones/ShutterStock, Inc.; Painting of houses
    © Aga & Miko (arsat)/ShutterStock, Inc.
Printing and Binding: Malloy Incorporated
Cover Printing: Malloy Incorporated

Library of Congress Cataloging-in-Publication Data
Family violence : what health care providers need to know/[edited by] Rose
S. Fife and Sarina Schrager.
   p. ; cm.
Includes bibliographical references and index.
ISBN 978-0-7637-8034-0
1. Family violence. I. Fife, Rose S. II. Schrager, Sarina B.
[DNLM: 1. Domestic Violence—prevention & control. 2. Battered
Women—psychology. 3. Crisis Intervention. 4. Mandatory Reporting. WA 308]
RC569.5.F3F373 2012
616.85'822—dc22
                              2010046745
6048
Printed in the United States of America
15 14 13 12 11   10 9 8 7 6 5 4 3 2 1

Contents

Chapter 5   **Bullying** **45**
by Sarina Schrager, MD, MS

Chapter 6   **Intimate Partner Violence** **51**
by DaWana Stubbs, MD, MS; Rose S. Fife, MD, MPH

Chapter 7   **Intimate Partner Violence and
Women's Reproductive Health** **59**
by Sarina Schrager, MD, MS

Acknowledgments

The editors are grateful to all of the contributors for their thoughtful, comprehensive chapters. We would also like to thank those who helped us find information or directed us to appropriate sources, such as Kathleen Grove, who brought several college programs on preventing dating violence to our attention, and the patients who shared with us the reality of living in a violent relationship. We would like to acknowledge the team at Jones & Bartlett Learning. Finally, we both want to thank our families for their patience and support through the time-consuming but highly rewarding process of creating this book.

Contributing Authors

Kerry Hyatt Blomquist, JD
Legal Director
Indiana Coalition Against Domestic Violence

Juliet Bradley, MD
Associate Professor of Clinical Medicine, Cook County
Loyola University Medical School
Family Medicine Residency Program
Provident Hospital of Cook County

Pamela L. Carter-Nolan, PhD, MPH
Assistant Dean for Medical Education
VP for Education (CFM)
Howard University College of Medicine

Lois S. Cronholm, PhD
Professor of Biology, Baruch College
Sr. Vice President, City University of New York (ret.)

Peter Cronholm, MD, MSCE
Assistant Professor, Department of Family Medicine
    and Community Health
Firearm & Injury Center at Pennsylvania
University of Pennsylvania

Ann M. Delaney, JD
The Julian Center, Inc.

Deborah Dreyfus, MD
Department of Family Medicine
Boston University

Valerie J. Gilchrist, MD
Department of Family Medicine
University of Wisconsin

Amy S. Gottlieb, MD
Assistant Professor of Medicine and Obstetrics and
    Gynecology (Clinical)
The Warren Alpert Medical School of Brown University
Director of Primary Care Curricula and Consultation
Internal Medicine Attending Physician, Women's
    Primary Care Center
Women & Infants Hospital

Judith A. Gravdal, MD
Advocate Lutheran General Hospital

Maren E. Hyde-Nolan, PhD
Doctors' Hospital of Michigan

Tracy Juliao, PhD
Family Medicine Residency
Doctor's Hospital of Michigan

Sandra Kamnetz, MD
UW Health–Monona

Tony Lapp, LCSW
Assistant Director
Menergy

Antoinette L. Laskey, MD, MPH
Associate Professor of Pediatrics
Children's Health Services Research

Charles P. Mouton, MD, MS
Meharry Medical College

Kathy Oriel, MD, MS
Department of Family Medicine
University of Wisconsin School of Medicine and Public Health

Mary Beth Plane, MSSW, PhD
Department of Family Medicine
University of Wisconsin

Jo Marie Reilly, MD
USC Keck School of Medicine

Anantha Shekhar, MD, PhD
Associate Dean for Translational Research
Indiana University School of Medicine

DaWana Stubbs, MD, MS
Assistant Professor of Medicine
Indiana University School of Medicine

Darlene D. West, DDS
Indiana University School of Dentistry

Betsy Whaley, MDiv
The Julian Center, Inc.

Karen M. Yoder, PhD
Indiana University School of Dentistry

Chapter 1

Introduction to Family Violence

Rose S. Fife, MD, MPH

INTRODUCTION

Our goals for this book are to provide you with a solid grounding in the field of family violence; to discuss as much as is known about incidence, prevalence, etiology, and management; and to provide a foundation through access to information and references for healthcare providers from all areas of medicine (i.e., physicians, nurses, dentists, social workers, allied health professionals) to recognize and to assist your patients with this all-too-common problem.

Family violence is a true public health epidemic in the United States and, indeed, in all parts of the world in which it has been examined. It crosses all socioeconomic, demographic, educational, and religious boundaries; it affects recent immigrants to the United States, as well as those whose ancestors arrived in the 17th century and before; it touches the rich and the poor, the well educated and the high school dropouts, the young and the old, males and females. Few discuss family violence in public because it is associated with much stigma; few healthcare providers can recognize it, and, if they do, they may not know what to do about it; few victims even report the violence. Sadly, the legal system, the social services sectors (both private and public), and families often do not recognize the problem or do not know how to deal with it. Indeed, the status of family abuse victims is similar to that of individuals with HIV/AIDS in the early 1980s when that disease was barely recognized, hardly discussed, highly stigmatized, and often ignored or denied. Fortunately, we have come a long way in our battle against HIV/AIDS in the last three decades. Sadly, we have made relatively little progress in our battle against family violence over the centuries.

Through this book, we want to do our part to increase awareness, recognition, discussion, and management of family violence. We want to help set the stage for those who follow to develop effective and facile programs to reduce and ultimately prevent this devastating epidemic.

DEFINITIONS

Family violence encompasses child abuse, intimate partner (or domestic) violence, and elder abuse. All of these forms of abuse can include verbal, psychological, physical, and sexual components. In many cases, they are interrelated, as we will show in subsequent chapters: People who have been abused as children are more likely to be abused as they grow older (see Chapters 2, 4, and 13). Similarly, perpetrators of violence are more likely to have been abused as children. Central to the causation of family violence, to the best of our knowledge, is the concept of control (See Chapters 2, 3, and 6): The abuser often feels the need to control all aspects of the victim's life, from what she can wear, to how much money, if any, she can access, to whom she may speak, to whether or not she can use the phone, leave the house, drive a car, and so on. (Please note that, although abusers can be male or female, the overwhelming majority of reported episodes of heterosexual abuse of any kind, beyond early adolescence, are male to female.) Some survivors were essentially imprisoned in their homes for years before they finally managed to leave their abusers. Many victims have had little or no contact with their families or friends for years, and many are accused and punished for things that they did not do.

STATISTICS

Due to the under-reporting and under-recognition of all aspects of family violence, the available numbers regarding its occurrence may not be accurate. However, the best estimates are that at least 20–30% of all females in the United States will be abused at some point during their lives. Most of the homicides of women are at the hands of an intimate partner or relative. Males, both heterosexual and homosexual, are also abused, but those numbers are even less accurate than for female victims. Abuse in lesbian relationships occurs too. As noted earlier and elsewhere in this book, family violence is an equal opportunity scourge, knowing no racial, ethnic, gender, age, religious, economic, or educational boundaries. In fact, most people know someone who has been abused, even if they are not aware that the abuse has occurred.

CONSEQUENCES

Aside from the obvious harm sustained by victims, family abuse affects all of society in some way. The estimated cost of all aspects of family violence is probably in the vicinity of $10–15 billion a year when medical care, days lost from work, criminal prosecution, social services, and loss of lifelong productivity as a result of trauma and death are included. The toll also includes long-term mental health disorders, such as increased post-traumatic stress disorder; increased cigarette, alcohol, and drug use; chronic health problems, such as obesity, pain, headaches; poor pregnancy outcomes; avoidance of interactions with healthcare providers; and inability to pay for care. Additionally, family violence can spill out of the home into the workplace, public transportation, schools, and other public sites, where the perpetrator often injures or kills others while attempting to harm his victim.

Another point that needs to be addressed is that the casual observer, the person who learns of someone else's abuse, often wonders why the victim did not leave as soon as the violence started. Even healthcare providers are subject to such pondering. Although it is well and good for people to suggest that a woman leave, it must be understood that typically she cannot do so immediately, and often not for a long time. There are many reasons for this: She may think this lifestyle is "normal"; she may have developed a variant of the Stockholm syndrome and identifies and agrees with the abuser that she is bad or stupid or deserves this; she may be so isolated from family and friends that she has no idea of how to leave or where to go; she may have no job skills and fear that she and her children will starve. Most importantly, though, she is probably scared of the consequences of leaving, possibly because her abuser has threatened her with statements like "If I can't have you nobody can," or "I'll kill you if you try to leave," or "I'll hunt you till I find you." These are valid fears because a woman's risk of being killed (and likewise of her children being wounded or killed) is highest when she tries to leave. As discussed elsewhere (Chapter 17), the construct of the Transtheoretical model of health behavior change developed by DiClemente and Prochaska[1] is consistent with this process: A woman must get to the point of recognizing the abuse, be ready to leave, and develop a plan for how to leave. Thus, although family, friends, healthcare providers, and others can and should help her leave, it should be when she is ready to do so and has a plan established that is as safe as possible. Harassing her with questions like "Why don't you leave that monster?" or "How can you stay there?" does not help her at all and may be dangerous in the short term.

THE WAY FORWARD

Clearly, much work must be done in all aspects of family violence: We must improve the ability of healthcare providers to recognize the signs of family violence, and increase their knowledge of how to approach and help victims; we must enable the legal system to identify, to prosecute, and to sentence perpetrators appropriately, and to protect the survivors; we must create effective and reproducible interventions that are age-appropriate, audience-appropriate, and proven to produce the desired outcome of reducing and ultimately eliminating family violence. Countless people have been working on family violence issues for many years, and therefore, we have no illusions about making any immediate breakthrough in these areas via this small book. However, we believe that the more information everybody has, the more people can work together to reduce this epidemic; the more that people work together, the more others will think about it, and eventually the reduction and ultimate elimination of family violence will come. We hope that a few of you who read this book may eventually develop some programs that help make the reduction and ultimate elimination come sooner.

REFERENCE

1. Prochaska JO, Velicer WF. The transtheoretical model of health behavior change. *Am J Health Promot.* 1997 Sep-Oct;12(1):38–48.

Chapter 2

Theoretical Basis for Family Violence

Maren E. Hyde-Nolan, PhD
Tracy Juliao, PhD

INTRODUCTION

A number of different psychological theories address the causes of family violence (FV). The most popular theories all acknowledge the abuse of power and control by the abusers, although the role of power and control varies by theoretical orientation. In this chapter, we focus on four main theoretical categories: (1) psychoanalytic theories of FV, (2) social theories of FV, (3) cognitive behavioral theories of FV, and (4) family and systems theories of FV. Psychoanalytic theories focus on individual internal psychological processes that create a need to be abusive or to accept abusive behavior. Social theories focus on how aggression, abuse, and violence are learned and transferred by individual members of the family to others within the family. Cognitive behavior theories also focus on how aggression, abuse, and violence are learned and transferred among individuals, but these theories further attempt to explain why abusive behaviors are sometimes transmitted from generation to generation while other times they are not. Finally, family and systems theories focus on the interactions between family members and the shared responsibility for the events that occur within the family system.

Some theories of FV have been left out of the review in this chapter, so we will briefly mention a few of them here. For instance, the feminist perspective regarding FV focuses on patriarchal societies that foster a patriarchal family structure in which men are expected to have power over women.[1]

Similarly, historical and ecological approaches to FV suggest that violence against women and children has always been present, noting that certain groups become targets within certain societies.[2] Finally, although there are various cultural theories of FV,[3-7] we have decided to conceptualize cultural considerations as an overarching umbrella under which all other theories of FV fall. In other words, it is impossible to understand FV in the absence of a cultural understanding of the individuals involved in the behaviors in question.

PSYCHODYNAMIC THEORIES OF FAMILY VIOLENCE

Three psychodynamic theories are discussed: object relations theory, attachment theory, and a theory called violence as trauma.

Object Relations Theory

Object relations theory suggests that humans are motivated from their earliest childhood by the need for significant relationships with others;[8] "others" are referred to as "objects" within objects relations theory. To reduce the potential for confusion, we simply refer to "objects" as "others" or "other individuals" in this chapter. Fairbairn[8] suggests that these early relationships, in addition to playing a role in psychic development, form the enduring psychological "templates" for all of the individual's future relationships. In essence, object relations theory proposes that individuals develop mental representations of themselves, other individuals, and the relationships between themselves and others beginning in infancy and childhood; these mental representations carry over and influence interpersonal relationships throughout life.[8-11] Many prominent object relations theorists suggest that the child's early experiences in his or her relationship with the primary caregiver set the stage for the development of stable, enduring, internalized mental representations of oneself, others, and the emotional experiences that are attached to the relationship between the oneself and others.[12-16]

The first years of life are extremely important for individuals to ensure the development of adequate emotional health in later life.[11] Individuals who lacked sufficient nurturing during infancy and childhood may find it difficult to maintain healthy self-esteem, regulate their emotional responses, and manage anxiety in later life. Unmet dependency needs in childhood persist into adulthood, often accompanied by a sense of rage that one's needs were not met. As a result, the search to fulfill dependency needs as an adult becomes both desperate and demanding,[1] which could lead to relationships in which one is either an abuser or a victim.[9,10,17,18] For example, evidence suggests that at least some men who commit intimate partner violence (IPV) did not receive adequate nurturing in the first years of development.[11,17] Dutton et al[18] found that becoming an adult perpetrator of IPV was significantly correlated with violence in the family of origin, as well as with parental rejection. In contrast, it has been argued that individuals who become victims of violence in adolescent and/or adult relationships, and who continue to maintain those relationships despite the violence, do so because of internal defenses that are employed during early development in an abusive, neglectful, or inconsistent relationship with the primary caregiver.[9,10,17] The development and utilization of defenses during infancy and childhood is highly adaptive, in that doing so allows for survival within an abusive family situation.[9] However, when these defenses are carried over into adolescent or adult relationships, they are maladaptive and prevent the individual from effectively recognizing the presence or absence of abuse in relationships and further promote maintenance of a relationship with someone who resembles the abusive primary caretaker from infancy and childhood.[9,10]

Attachment Theory

Unlike the emphasis placed on the individual's mental representation of a relationship in the object relations theory, attachment theory emphasizes reciprocity between individuals within a relationship. Attachment is defined as a reciprocal, enduring emotional tie between an infant and a caregiver, with both parties actively contributing to the quality of the relationship.[19] According to the early attachment theorists, Bowlby[20] and Ainsworth,[21] an infant develops a "working model" of what can be expected from his or her primary caregiver. If the caregiver continues to respond in expected ways, the infant's model holds up; however, if the caregiver's responses become consistently unpredictable, the infant is forced to revise his or her model, and the security of the attachment changes.[21] The basic concept underlying the theory of attachment is that adults have the power to both protect and provide a sense of security for their children. At times when the child feels threatened, exhausted, or ill, he or she will turn to the caregiver for security and protection.[22] Once the attachment bond is formed, it ensures that the secure base of the relationship is in place. One of the key features of such a secure base is the relationship between security and exploration. A child with secure attachment can explore the environment, but when the child feels threatened, attachment behaviors are activated, and the child will seek out the secure caregiver.[22] Children build a representation of their own worthiness based on their experiences and perceptions of the caregiver's ability, availability, and willingness to provide care and protection.[23] Over time the child is able to use the symbolic representations of important attachment figures to feel secure without the presence of the caregiver. However, not all attachments are positive. Although secure attachments are preferred and most common (60–75%), avoidant, ambivalent, and disorganized/disoriented attachments can also develop within parent–child relationships that are less predictable.[19]

Attachment theory explains that child abuse results in insecure and anxious attachment, which can be avoidant, ambivalent, or disorganized.[24] Anxious attachment can be viewed as a marker for later social and emotional problems and is most likely to occur in situations of maltreatment.[25] Unfortunately, distorted patterns of relating to others lay the foundation for the child's model of the world, influence how the child responds, and may prevent the child from developing a positive internal model of self.[26,27] Research findings suggest that antisocial behavior may be linked with early adverse family experiences, especially with patterns of insecure attachment.[28,29] Several studies also have shown that insecure attachment occurs more often in populations of children who have experienced physical abuse or neglect.[30–34] Moreover, attachment theory may explain the perpetuation of child maltreatment from one generation to the next.[35]

Violence as Trauma

The theory of violence as trauma has contributed a great deal to our understanding of how an individual incorporates internal defenses into his or her personality structure[36–39] and has clarified how those defenses affect interpersonal relationships.[36,38,40,41]

The theory of violence as trauma suggests that victims of abuse process this experience as a traumatic event, much like the response of individuals who suffer from post-traumatic stress disorder.[42–44] It is important to understand how an individual victim processed the information of the trauma into memory because the trauma may affect the way in which future information is processed, including how events are coded, stored, and sequenced.[45] Trauma also may disrupt how information is managed because sensory stimuli enter the brain's limbic system.[46] When the limbic system is overridden due to high levels of stress and trauma, the inability to handle the stressors can cause the individual to switch to survival techniques known as psychological numbing.[46]

The psychobiology of post-traumatic stress offers an explanation for why victims of abuse seem to experience abusive situations repeatedly. These individuals appear to have a compulsion to repeat the trauma due to the inability to integrate their memories of abuse, as well as to incorporate their abusive experiences, into their larger memory structure.[47] In this model, the trauma is repeated emotionally, behaviorally, physiologically, and via the neuroendocrine (i.e., fight-or-flight patterns) pathways for abused individuals.[47] In this theory, victims of abuse emotionally repeat the trauma by aligning themselves with people who will continue to abuse them in some way. They repeat the trauma behaviorally through repetition, re-enactment, and displacement of the abusive experience.[45] In addition, victims physiologically continue the trauma by re-experiencing the bodily memory of the abuse, most often in the form of pain.[46] The traumatic replay of an abusive event in the memory releases chemicals in the brain that override the fight-or-flight system.[47] As a result, victims remain vulnerable to further situations of abuse because they are unable to defend themselves.[48]

SOCIAL THEORIES OF FAMILY VIOLENCE

The social theories of FV focus on processes that are created via interactions with others in one-to-one relationships or in larger groups. Four social theories are discussed: control theory, resource theory, exosystem factor theory, and social isolation theory.

Control Theory

Control theory is based on the concept that many family conflicts result from an individual's need to obtain and maintain power and control within a relationship(s). The motivation underlying the abuser's behavior is the power and control that she or he is able to exert over other members of the family.[49] The more powerful members of families (e.g., fathers, parents, husbands) often use the threat or use of force or the threat or use of violence to obtain compliance from less powerful family members (e.g., children, wives).[50] Threats, force, and violent behaviors are intended to prohibit the less powerful members of the family from engaging in behavior that the controlling individual does not want, while establishing a demand for "desirable" behaviors to occur.[50] In addition, the abuser may feel the need to gain control over how other family members think and feel.[49] Abusers, in an effort to maintain control over other members of the family, may use many forms of intimidation, such as coercion, isolation, economic abuse, and denial of personal blame.[49] The victim(s) typically learn how to respond to the various forms of intimidation, although the struggle to challenge the abuse/abuser may become too overwhelming or dangerous for the victim(s). As a result, the victim(s) may begin to modify his/her/their own behavior, slowly giving up control in order to survive and avoid continued abuse. Isolating the victim from any social contacts may be the most harmful form of intimidation the abuser uses because the possibility of escape for the victim(s) is greatly reduced in the absence of social support.[49]

In addition to seeking to explain why some family members are violent, control theory also seeks to explain why other people are *not* violent.[51] Whereas some individuals are desperate to obtain power, others are controlled by the fear of punishment, as well as their bonds to other people and/or institutions. In fact, research in FV has discovered that men who have strong attachments to significant others and fear negative reactions from these individuals are less likely to abuse their wives than men without these attachments.[52] Similarly, men who value attachments to home, work, and community may view the threat of arrest for spousal abuse as a significant disincentive from engaging in such behavior.[53]

Resource Theory

Resource theory suggests a relationship between wealth and violence.[50] This theory proposes that force and violence are resources that can be used to resolve conflicts, although in modern society these resources are often used as a last resort.[50] For example, men with high income and social standing have access to a wide variety of resources with which to control their wives' behavior (in addition to violence), whereas men with limited or no wealth and resources may resort to physical force or violence more quickly.[54]

Exosystem Factor Theory

Exosystem factor theory also includes the notion of the importance of resources. This theory focuses on life stressors, which are considered to be specific life events or experiences that are perceived by the individual as exceeding his or her resources.[55] According to this theory, stressors, or life events, can serve as predictors of FV. Stressors/life events may include experiences such as job loss, an extramarital affair, moving to a new home, or daily hassles such as traffic and paying bills. There may be a direct relationship between husband-to-wife violence and the perception and frequency of stressors.[56]

Stress results in FV only when other specific factors are present, including a personal history of growing up in a violent family, low marital satisfaction, and social isolation.[55,57] Violence is only one of many possible stress responses, however.[55] For example, despite the evidence of a positive association between number of stressors experienced in a year and the rate of child abuse, a number of intervening variables also play a role in the relationship.[57] Stress is related to child abuse among individuals who had learned to use violence during childhood and who also believed that hitting family members was justified.[55] However, when these factors were not present, the relationship between stress and abuse was minimal. Therefore, stress is an important but not essential factor for predicting FV.[55]

Social Isolation Theory

Social isolation has been identified as an intervening variable between stressors/life events and FV.[55] Social isolation theory posits that child abuse and neglect are associated with isolation of the parent–child relationship from social support systems.[58] Based on this perspective, understanding child maltreatment requires looking beyond high-risk families to neighborhoods and larger systems that have higher rates of child maltreatment. Garbarino and Sherman[59] studied communities that were matched on socioeconomic status (SES) and race, but had differing rates of reported child maltreatment. They found that in high-risk neighborhoods, family problems were considerably worse when families were isolated rather than part of a community. A subsequent study of communities in the Chicago area indicated that the areas with the highest rates of child maltreatment had greater social disorganization in the form of crime, along with a lack of availability of social services and support networks and minimal to no knowledge regarding the resources that do exist.[60]

COGNITIVE/BEHAVIORAL THEORIES OF FAMILY VIOLENCE

Cognitive and behavioral theories focus on individual-level factors that contribute to FV. In this section, four cognitive/behavioral theories are discussed: social learning theory, behavior genetics theory, the theory of reactive aggression, and the theory of learned helplessness.

Social Learning Theory

Social learning theory maintains that individuals learn social behaviors by observing and imitating other people.[61,62] Imitation of models is the most important element in how children learn. This process can be seen in the development of language, aggression, and moral decision-making.[19] Social learning theory posits that individuals become aggressive toward family members because their aggressive behaviors are learned through operant conditioning and observing behavior in role models.[55] Operant conditioning is the strengthening of behaviors through positive and negative reinforcement, as well as the suppression of behaviors through punishment.[55] In fact, corporal punishment may be chosen as a discipline method simply because it typically brings about children's compliance with parental demands.[63] However, research points to both short- and long-term negative effects associated with physical punishment, such as increased physical aggressiveness, antisocial behavior, poor parent–child relationships during childhood,[63,64] and aggression, criminal behavior, mental health problems, and partner or spousal abuse in adulthood.[63,65]

Social learning theory attempts to explain the presence of intergenerational transmission of violence. It is proposed that, while growing up, children receive feedback from others regarding their own behaviors, from which they begin to develop standards for judging their behavior and seek out models who match these standards.[62] Children who grow up in violent/abusive families may learn violent/abusive behaviors, imitate those behaviors, and then repeat those behaviors in future relationships. Several studies have indicated that individuals who were abused in childhood are at greater risk for abusing their own children in adulthood.[66,67] In addition, men who observed their fathers abusing their mothers when they were children are at an increased risk for abusing their wives.[68,69] Finally, researchers have found that young adults who observed and experienced abuse when they were children are more likely to be in an abusive intimate relationship as either abuser or victim.[70,71]

Behavioral Genetics

Behavioral genetics theory posits that genetic factors, in addition to factors associated with social learning, may explain the similarities found among family members and their use of violence.[72] A review of the behavioral genetics literature demonstrated that the characteristics of aggression and antisocial behavior seem to be genetically influenced.[72] Although individuals may have a genetic predisposition toward engaging in aggressive behavior, the form of aggression they engage in will vary based on differences in non-shared environmental influences, such as stress and exposure to violence. Both heredity and environment impact the perpetuation of FV from one generation to the next.[72,73]

Reactive Aggression

The theory of reactive aggression focuses on emotional and cognitive processes leading to behavioral responses. This theory posits that the following events occur when an individual experiences an unpleasant situation:

(1) an aversive stimulus results in a negative emotional response, (2) the negative emotional response then leads to an urge to hurt others or thoughts of hurting others, and (3) the urge to hurt results in aggressive behavior unless inhibiting factors are present.[74]

The theory of reactive aggression has been suggested in FV in several studies. Some researchers have described a positive correlation between parental self-reports of anger and the use of physical discipline with their children, as well as the risk for child abuse in their families.[75] In addition, one study classified a group of men who abuse their spouses as "borderline/cyclical batterers."[76] These men have been observed to react with rage when they perceive or are faced with actual rejection or abandonment by their spouses. Once these men experience emotional pain, they are overcome with the desire to hurt, and thoughts about hurting, their spouses. The desire and thoughts may be immediately followed by rage and violent behaviors toward their spouses unless something happens to derail them (e.g., arrival of the police in response to a call from a neighbor or a knock on the door from an unexpected visitor). The reaction to aggress when faced with situations of pain and anger aids in our understanding of why FV occurs and may increase our ability to combat the cognitive distortions that underlie some of the aggressive and abusive behaviors in which individuals engage, as explained by this theory.

Learned Helplessness

The theory of learned helplessness sheds light on reasons why victims of FV often choose to stay in somewhat unpredictable and volatile family relationships. The theory of learned helplessness was originally proposed to explain the loss of will that accompanies repeated barriers to escape from an aversive situation.[77] By chance, while studying depression in experiments with dogs, Seligman[77] discovered that sometimes dogs would "learn" that their behaviors did not bring about the expected or desired outcome in situations where barriers (electric shock) were present. As a result, the dogs would stop engaging in the behavior even once the barriers were removed. Much like the dogs that "learned" to be helpless after being subjected to electric shocks with no ability to escape, battered women may fall into the same pattern.[78] Experiencing repeated beatings or other abuse may lead a woman to become passive because she feels that nothing she does will result in a positive outcome. This theory of violence is controversial because many women in a violent relationship do maintain a sense of dignity, learn skills to survive, and may even fight back.[79]

FAMILY AND SYSTEMS THEORIES OF FAMILY VIOLENCE

Family and systems theories focus on the family unit and attempt to explain individual behaviors within the context of interpersonal relationships, family systems, and larger societal systems, as well as how these relate to the formation and maintenance of FV.

Three family and system theories are discussed in detail: family systems theory, family life cycle theory, and microsystem factor theories (including the sub-theories of intrafamilial stress and dependency relations). The cycle of violence theory is one of the most popular theories for explaining FV and is described in full detail in Chapter 3.

Family Systems Theory

Family systems theory is based on the idea that each individual should be viewed not in isolation but in terms of the interactions, transitions, and relationships within the family.[80] The focus of assessment and intervention shifts from one individual to the patterns of relationships among all individuals in a family group.[81] A central tenet of this theory is that what affects one individual affects the entire family system and what affects the family system affects each member as well.[82] Family systems theory provides a framework for observing and understanding general characteristics of human relationships, individual functioning within the nuclear family, ways in which emotional problems are transmitted to the next generation, as well as the transmission of behavioral patterns over multiple generations, which is particularly important when attempting to understand FV.[83] Additionally, it is important to remember that the family system is a sub-system within larger systems, such as the community,[81] which interact with and influence one another and contribute to the maintenance of particular patterns of behavior.

Family Life Cycle Theory

The family life cycle theory posits that, to understand families, we must examine transitions in the family experience. At its early inception, family life cycle theorists divided family development into discrete stages, with specific tasks to be performed at each stage.[84,85] These stages tend to coincide with family members entering and exiting due to marriage, death, the addition of a child, or a young adult leaving the parental home.[82] Carter and McGoldrick[86] expanded this model to include a multigenerational point of view, as well as a cultural perspective. They suggested that the family life cycle includes approximately six stages: single young adulthood, joining of families (the new couple), families with young children, families with adolescents, families launching children and moving on, and families in later life. Family life cycle theory adds two important concepts to our understanding of individual development, which might aid in understanding how and why FV occurs and is often repeated: (1) families often must reorganize to accommodate the growth and change of their members, and (2) development in any generation of the family may have an impact on one or all of the family's members.[81]

However, although many variations of lifestyles, family formations, and behaviors exist, it is important to note that life cycle transitions of any form can result in stress experienced by the family system. Changes in life cycle stages are critical transition points for families and their individual members.[84–86] When a family system is inflexible and unable to adapt and maintain balance between stability and change, it may become dysfunctional.[82] In addition, the stress that results from life cycle transitions can lead to violence within the family system. In fact, the most dangerous time in a FV relationship occurs during marital/partner separation when serious physical harm or death is more likely to occur.[2]

Microsystem Factor Theories

FV and abuse also have been conceptualized in terms of an ecological model that includes causes within the family unit and causes that pertain to cultural factors and any systemic factor in between.[87,88] Microsystem factor theories place emphasis on stresses that inherently exist within the family as a social structure. The microsystem consists of the interactions between the developing individual and the immediate settings (e.g., home, school) where the individual interacts with others.[55] The two microsystem factor theories that are discussed next are intrafamilial stress theory and dependency relations theory.

Intrafamilial Stress Theory

Intrafamilial stress includes factors such as having more children than the parents can afford, overcrowded living conditions, and having children with disabilities.[55] This theory posits that these situations can place a significant burden on the family system, particularly in terms of time and resources, which may contribute to violent behavior. The ecological perspective indicates that intrafamilial stress and beliefs regarding parenting also may interact. For instance, the association between parental stress and the risk of child abuse varies as a result of the parent's belief in implementing corporal punishment.[89]

Dependency Relations Theory

Dependency relations theory is based on the concept that victims of abuse are dependent on their abusers (which is not true in some situations). The role of dependency in FV has been found in child, elder, and spousal abuse.[90] Children remain dependent on their abusers because they tend to be smaller and weaker than adults and are unable to escape from an abusive family or violent neighborhood or support themselves. Some elderly become frail, sick, dependent, and difficult to care for, which results in stress for their caregivers and dependency on their abusers.[90,91] Even some well-meaning caretakers, who are most often relatives, may lose control when under stress and become abusive toward their elderly family members.[91] Additionally, like children, some older people may become dependent on family members for basic care, which may be a risk factor for abuse.[92] In spousal abuse, economic dependency may be a reason that explains why many women stay in abusive marriages.[93] Maltreated wives may have little or no income of their own and thus may believe that they would not be able to support themselves or their children if they were to leave the abusive relationship.[93] Dependence may be exacerbated in immigrant women who may be afraid of being alone in a foreign country and also may fear bringing perceived shame on their families if they were to divorce their abusers (Chapter 10).[94]

Although this chapter has provided an overview of some theories that are thought to help explain the development, existence, and maintenance of FV, no single theory in and of itself is likely sufficient to explain this phenomenon. Complex behaviors, complicated thinking patterns, individual psychologies, and the interactions among individuals and systems all can play a role in FV.

REFERENCES

1. Bograd M. Power, gender and the family: feminist perspectives on family systems therapy. In: Dutton-Douglas MA, Walker LEA, eds. *Feminist Psychotherapies: Integration of Therapeutic and Feminist Systems.* Norwood, NJ: Ablex; 1988:118–133.
2. Walker LEA. Assessment of abusive spousal relationships. In: Kaslow FW, ed. *Handbook of Relational Diagnosis and Dysfunctional Family Patterns.* New York, NY: Wiley; 1996.
3. Boyd-Franklin N. *Black Families in Therapy: A Multisystems Approach.* New York, NY: Guildford Press; 1989.
4. Flores MT, Carey G. *Family Therapy with Hispanics: Toward Appreciating Diversity.* Boston, MA: Allyn & Bacon; 2000.
5. McGoldrick M, Giordano J, Pearce JK. *Ethnicity and Family Therapy.* 2nd ed. New York, NY: Guilford Press; 1996.

6. Minuchin P, Colapinto J, Minuchin S. *Working with Families of the Poor.* New York, NY: Guilford Press; 1998.

7. Walters M, Carter B, Papp P, Silverstein O. *The Invisible Web: Gender Patterns in Family Relationships.* New York, NY: Guilford Press; 1988.

8. Fairbairn WRD. *An Object Relations Theory of the Personality.* London, United Kingdom: Tavistock; 1952.

9. Blizard RA, Bluhn AM. Attachment to the abuser: Integrating object relations and trauma theories in treatment of abuse survivors. *Psychotherapy.* 1994; 31(3):383–390.

10. Cogan R, Porcerelli JH, Dromgoole K. Psychodynamics of partner, stranger, and generally violent male college students. *Psychoanal Psychol.* 2001;18:513–33.

11. Zosky DL. The application of object relations theory to domestic violence. *Clin Soc Work J.* 1999;27:55–69.

12. Kernberg OF. *Object Relations Theory and Clinical Psychoanalysis.* Northvale, NJ: Jason Aronson; 1984.

13. Kernberg OF. *Internal World and External Reality: Objects Relations Theory Applied.* Northvale, NJ: Jason Aronson; 1985.

14. Kernberg OF. *Severe Personality Disorders: Psychotherapeutic Strategies.* New Haven, CT: Yale University Press; 1986.

15. Masterson JF. *Psychotherapy of the Borderline Adult: A Developmental Approach.* New York, NY: Brunner/Mazel; 1976.

16. Masterson JF. *The Narcissistic and Borderline Disorders: An Integrated Developmental Approach.* New York, NY: Brunner/Mazel; 1981.

17. Cogan R, Porcerelli JH. Object relations in abusive partner relationships: An empirical investigation. *J Pers Assess.* 1996;66:105–115.

18. Dutton DG, Starzomski A, Ryan L. Antecedents of abusive personality and abusive behavior in wife assaulters. *J Fam Violence.* 1996;11:113–132.

19. Papalia DE, Olds SW, Feldman RD. *Human Development.* 11th ed. Boston, MA: McGraw-Hill; 2010.

20. Bowlby J. Maternal care and mental health. *Bull World Health Organ.* 1951;3:355–534.

21. Ainsworth MDS. *Infancy in Uganda: Infant Care and the Growth of Love.* Baltimore, MD: Johns Hopkins University Press; 1967.

22. Holmes J. Attachment theory and abuse: A developmental perspective. In: McCluskey U, Hooper C, eds. *Psychodynamic Perspectives on Abuse: The Cost of Fear.* London, United Kingdom: Jessica Kingsley; 2000:40–53.

23. Bowlby J. *Separation: Anxiety and Anger.* Harmondsworth, United Kingdom: Penguin; 1973. *Attachment and Loss;* vol 2.

24. Crittenden PM, Ainsworth M. Child maltreatment and attachment theory. In: Cicchetti D, Carlson V, eds. *Child Maltreatment, Theory and Research on the Causes and Consequences of Child Abuse and Neglect.* New York, NY: Cambridge University Press; 1989.

25. Lewis M, Feiring C, McGuffog C, Jaskir J. Predicting psychopathology in six-year olds from early social relations. *Child Dev.* 1984;55:123–136.

26. Bowlby J. On knowing what you are not supposed to know and feeling what you are not supposed to feel. In: Bowlby J, ed. *A Secure Base.* London, United Kingdom: Routledge; 1988.

27. Crittenden PM. Family and dyadic patterns of functioning in maltreatment. In: Browne K, Davies C, Stratton P, eds. *Early Prediction and Prevention of Child Abuse.* Chichester, United Kingdom: Wiley; 1988.

28. Cicchetti D, Lynch M. Towards an ecological/transactional model of community violence and child maltreatment: consequences for children's development. *Psychiatry.* 1993;56:96–118.

29. Smallbone SW, Dadds MR. Attachment and coercive sexual behavior. *Sex Abuse.* 2000;12(1):3–15.

30. Bowlby J. Violence in the family as a disorder of the attachment and caregiving systems. *Am J Psychoanal.* 1984;44(1):9–27.

31. Carlson V, Cicchetti D, Barnett D, Braunwald K. Disorganized/disoriented attachment relationships in maltreated infants. *Dev Psychol.* 1989;25:525–531.

32. Dutton DG, Painter S. Traumatic bonding: the development of emotional attachments in battered women and other relationships of intermittent abuse. *Victimology.* 1991;6:139–155.

33. Lyons-Ruth K, Connell D, Zoll D. Patterns of maternal behavior among infants at risk for abuse: relations with infant attachment behavior and infant development at 12 months of age. In: Cicchetti D, Carlson V, eds. *Child Maltreatment, Theory and Research on the Causes and Consequences of Child Abuse and Neglect.* New York, NY: Cambridge University Press; 1989.

34. Main M, Goldwyn R. Predicting rejection of her infant from mother's representation of her own experience: implications for the abused–abuser intergenerational cycle. *Int J Child Abuse Negl.* 1984;8:203–217.

35. Morton N, Brown KD. Theory and observation of attachment and its relationship to child maltreatment: a review. *Child Abuse Negl.* 1998;22:1093–1105.

36. Fine CG. The cognitive sequelae of incest. In: Kluft RP, ed. *Incest-Related Syndromes of Adult Psychopathology.* Washington, DC: American Psychiatric Press; 1990.

37. Herman JL, van der Kolk BA. Traumatic antecedents of borderline personality disorder. In van der Kolk BA, ed. *Psychological Trauma.* Washington, DC: American Psychiatric Press; 1987.

38. Landecker H. The role of childhood sexual trauma in the etiology of borderline personality: considerations for diagnosis and treatment. *Psychotherapy.* 1992;29(2):234–242.

39. Rieker PR, Carmen EH. The victim-to-patient process: the disconfirmation and transformation of abuse. *Am J Orthopsychiatry.* 1986;56(3):360–369.

40. Gunderson JG, Sabo AN. The phenomenological and conceptual interface between borderline personality disorder and PTSD. *Am J Psychiatry.* 1993;150:19–27.

41. Kluft RP. Clinical presentations of multiple personality disorder. *Psychiatr Clin North Am.* 1991;14(3):605–630.

42. Putnam FW. *Diagnosis and Treatment of Multiple Personality Disorder.* New York, NY: Guildford; 1989.

43. Spiegel D. Multiple personality as a post-traumatic stress disorder. *Psychiatr Clin North Am.* 1984;7:101–110.

44. van der Kolk BA, Perry JC, Herman JL. Childhood origins of self-destructive behavior. *Am J Psychiatry.* 1991;149(12):1665–1671.

45. Burgess AW, Hartman CR, Kelley SJ. *Assessing Child Abuse: The TRIADS Checklist.* Instructional handout sheet presented at: Forensics Mental Health conference; 1990; Tampa, FL.

46. Brown SL. *Counseling Victims of Violence.* Alexandria, VA: American Association for Counseling and Development; 1991.

47. van der Kolk BA. The trauma spectrum: the interaction of biological and social events in the genesis of the trauma response. *J Traumatic Stress.* 1990;1:273–290.

48. van der Kolk BA, Greenberg MS, Boyd H, Krystal J. Inescapable shock, neuro-transmitters and addiction to trauma: toward a psychobiology of post-traumatic stress. *Biol Psychiatry.* 1985;20:314–325.

49. Bostock DJ, Auster S, Bradshaw RD, Brewster A, Chapin M, Williams C. Family violence. *American Academy of Family Physicians Home Study Self-Assessment Program* (Serial No. 274); 2002.

50. Goode WJ. Force and violence in the family. *J Marriage Fam.* 1971;33:624–636.

51. Loseke D. Through a sociological lens: the complexities of family violence. In: Loseke D, Gelles R, Cavanaugh M, eds. *Current Controversies on Family Violence.* 2nd ed. Thousand Oaks, CA: Sage; 2005.

52. Lackey C, Williams KR. Social bonding and the cessation of partner violence across generations. *J Marriage Fam.* 1995;57:295–305.

53. Sherman LW. *Policing Domestic Violence: Experiments and Dilemmas.* New York, NY: Free Press; 1992.

54. Anderson KL. Gender, status, and domestic violence: an integration of feminist and family violence approaches. *J Marriage Fam.* 1997;59:655–669.

55. Malley-Morrison K, Hines DA. *Family Violence in a Cultural Perspective: Defining, Understanding, and Combating Abuse.* Thousand Oaks, CA: Sage; 2004.

56. Cano A, Vivian D. Life stressors and husband-to-wife violence. *Aggression Violent Behav.* 2001;6:459–480.

57. Straus MA. Stress and physical child abuse. *Child Abuse Negl.* 1980;4:75–88.

58. Garbarino J. The human ecology of child maltreatment. *J Marriage Fam.* 1977;39:721–736.

59. Garbarino J, Sherman D. High-risk neighborhoods and high-risk families: the human ecology of child maltreatment. *Child Dev.* 1980;51:188–198.

60. Garbarino J, Kostelny K. Child maltreatment as a community problem. *Child Abuse Negl.* 1992;16:455–464.

61. Bandura A. *Social Learning Theory.* Englewood Cliffs, NJ: Prentice-Hall; 1977.

62. Bandura A. Social cognitive theory. In: Vasta R, ed. *Annals of Child Development.* Greenwich, CT: JAI; 1989.

63. Gershoff ET. Corporal punishment by parents and associated child behaviors and experiences: a meta-analytic and theoretical review. *Psychol Bull.* 2002;128:539–579.

64. Straussberg Z, Dodge KA, Pettit GS, Bates JE. Spanking in the home and chil-dren's subsequent aggression toward kindergarten peers. *Dev Psychopathol.* 1994;6:445–461.

65. MacMillan HM, Boyle MH, Wong MY-Y, Duku EK, Fleming JE, Walsh CA. Slapping and spanking in childhood and its association with lifetime prevalence of psychiatric disorders in a general population sample. *Can Med Assoc J.* 1999;161:805–809.

66. Jackson S, Thompson RA, Christiansen EH, et al. Predicting abuse-prone parental attitudes and discipline practices in a nationally representative sample. *Child Abuse Negl.* 1999;23:15–29.

67. Kaufman J, Zigler E. Do abused children become abusive parents? *Am J Orthopsychiatry.* 1987;57:186–192.

68. Corvo K, Carpenter E. Effects of parental substance abuse on current levels of domestic violence: a possible elaboration of intergenerational transmission processes. *J Fam Violence.* 2000;15:123–137.

69. Dutton DG. Male abusiveness in intimate relationships. *Clin Psychol Rev.* 1995;15:567–581.

70. Cappell C, Heiner RB. The intergenerational transmission of family aggression. *J Fam Violence.* 1990;5:135–152.

71. Marshall LL, Rose P. Premarital violence: the impact of family of origin on violence, stress, and reciprocity. *Violence Victims.* 1990;5:51–64.

72. Hines DA, Saudino KJ. Intergenerational transmission of intimate partner violence: a behavioral genetic perspective. *Trauma Violence Abuse.* 2002;3:210–225.

73. Saudino KJ, Hines DA. Etiological similarities between psychological and physical aggression in intimate relationships: a behavioral genetic exploration. *J Fam Violence.* 2007;22:121–129.

74. Berkowitz L. The goals of aggression. In: Finkelhor D, Gelles RJ, Hotaling GT, Straus MA, eds. *The Dark Side of Families: Current Family Violence Research.* Beverly Hills, CA: Sage; 1983:166–181.

75. Whiteman M, Fanshel D, Grundy JF. Cognitive-behavioral interventions aimed at anger of parents at risk of child abuse. *Soc Work.* 1987;32:469–474.

76. Douglas KS, Dutton DG. Assessing the link between stalking and domestic violence. *Aggression Violent Behav.* 2001;6:519–546.

77. Seligman M. *Helplessness: On Depression, Development, and Death.* New York, NY: W. H. Freeman; 1975.

78. Walker LE. *The Battered Woman.* New York, NY: Harper & Row; 1979.

79. Downs DA, Fisher J. Battered woman syndrome: tool of justice or false hope in self-defense cases? In: Loseke D, Gelles R, Cavanaugh M, eds. *Current Controversies on Family Violence.* 2nd ed. Thousand Oaks, CA: Sage; 2005.

80. Gurman AS, Kniskern DP. *Handbook of Family Therapy.* Vol 1. New York: NY: Brunner/Mazel; 1981.

81. Nichols MP, Schwartz RC. *Family Therapy: Concepts and Methods.* 6th ed. Boston, MA: Pearson/Allyn & Bacon; 2004.

82. McBride JL. Family behavioral issues. *American Academy of Family Physicians Home Study Self-Assessment Program* (Serial No. 285); 2003.

83. Bowen M. *Family Therapy in Clinical Practice.* Northvale, NJ: Jason Aronson; 1992.

84. Duvall E. *Family Development.* Philadelphia, PA: Lippincott; 1957.

85. Hill R, Rodgers R. The developmental approach. In: Christiansen HT, ed. *Handbook of Marriage and the Family.* Chicago, IL: Rand McNally; 1964.

86. Carter EA, McGoldrick M, eds. *The Expanded Family Life Cycle: Individual, Family, and Social Perspectives.* 3rd ed. Boston, MA: Allyn & Bacon; 1999.

87. Garbarino J. The consequences of child maltreatment: biosocial and ecological issues. In: Gelles RJ, Lancaster J, eds. *Child Abuse and Neglect.* Hawthorne, NY: Aldine de Gruyter; 1987:200–325.

88. Heise LL. Violence against women: an integrated, ecological framework. *Violence Against Women.* 1998;4:262–290.

89. Crouch JL, Behl LE. Relationships among parental beliefs in corporal punishment, reported stress, and physical child abuse potential. *Child Abuse Negl.* 2001;25:413–419.

90. Finkelhor D, Dziuba-Leatherman J. Victimization of children. *Am Psychologist.* 1994;49:173–183.

91. Pillemer K. Abuse is caused by the deviance and dependence of abusive caregivers. In: Loseke D, Gelles R, Cavanaugh M, eds. *Current Controversies on Family Violence.* 2nd ed. Thousand Oaks, CA: Sage; 1993.

92. Steinmetz SK. The abused elderly are dependent: abuse is caused by the perception of stress associated with providing care. In: Loseke D, Gelles R, Cavanaugh M, eds. *Current Controversies on Family Violence.* 2nd ed. Thousand Oaks, CA: Sage; 2005.

93. Wallace H. *Family Violence: Legal, Medical, and Social Perspectives.* 3rd ed. Boston, MA: Allyn & Bacon; 2002.

94. Dasgupta SD. Women's realities: defining violence against women by immigration, race, and class. In: Bergen RK, ed. *Issues in Intimate Violence.* Thousand Oaks, CA: Sage; 1998:209–219.

Chapter 3

The Cycle of Violence

Sarina Schrager, MD, MS

INTRODUCTION

The cycle of violence theory, described by Lenore Walker in her 1979 book, *The Battered Woman,* attempts to describe a pattern of behavior within an abusive intimate partner relationship.[1] The theory is based on interviews that Walker did with women who were in violent relationships. She interviewed 120 women in depth and more than 300 in some capacity. In her book, she uses the qualitative data from her interviews to develop a description of common attributes of abusive relationships. Although many have criticized this theory as not categorizing all abusive relationships, it has resonated with victims and violence prevention experts for the past 30 years and is included in most literature on violent intimate partner relationships.

The term *cycle of violence* also describes the relationship between violence experienced in childhood and future violent behavior in adulthood. Children who witness intimate partner violence are more likely to become victims as adults and have longer term psychological issues. Women who are victims of intimate partner violence (IPV) are more likely to become abused elders later in life.[2] This complex relationship is described elsewhere in this book.

Most relationships begin on a positive note, before any abuse starts, during which the couple "falls in love." Abuse in a relationship can begin at any point, but frequently does not start immediately after the beginning of the relationship. The actual cycle of abuse begins with a phase in which there is an escalation of tension and pressure between partners.

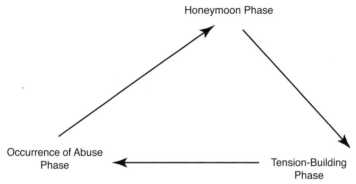

Figure 3–1 The cycle of violence.

The cycle of violence theory describes three distinct phases within a violent relationship (Figure 3–1): (1) the tension-building phase, (2) the occurrence of abuse, and (3) the honeymoon phase.

THE TENSION-BUILDING PHASE

This phase represents the beginning of the cycle. The beginning of a relationship (or during the first cycle) is a time when the victim is confronted by the new behavior of control by the abuser. In subsequent cycles, this phase is devastating for the victim because it may become apparent that things are not different this time and that the abusive pattern will continue. Many victims remain in denial and hope that each cycle is the last. The abuser becomes more irritable and unpredictable in his or her behavior. Minor incidents or disagreements that would be easy to resolve in the honeymoon phase become more serious. The victim tries to appease the abuser, not knowing what will trigger a violent outburst. Many have described the victim's behavior as "walking on eggshells," trying to be careful not to anger the abuser. The unpredictability is very stressful for the victim. In this phase, there is often escalating emotional abuse, threats, and intimidation by the abuser. There may be minor physical abuse toward the end of this phase leading up to the next phase in the cycle: occurrence of a major episode of abuse. The victim is continually afraid of what is going to happen next. In subsequent cycles of this pattern, the victim spends the tension-building phase anticipating a major episode of abuse. Many victims say that the anxiety over a future episode of violence is almost worse than the violence itself.

THE ABUSE PHASE

This phase is the culmination of the cycle of violence, when the tension of the abuser has grown to such a level that it must be released. The abuser explodes with a violent outburst. For the victim, the abuse feels like an inevitable conclusion of the cycle. The abuse is often a major physical attack by the abuser. The abuse can also be sexual, forcible restraint, or an escalation of emotional abuse. In this phase, the victim may try to leave, to protect himself or herself and their children, and do whatever is necessary to survive the episode of violence.

THE HONEYMOON PHASE

The honeymoon phase begins after the incident of serious abuse. This is the time in the relationship when everything is "back to normal." The abuser treats the victim well and can be very charming. The abuser apologizes for the abuse, promising it will never happen again. In subsequent cycles, this is the time when the victim is charmed by the abuser and decides to stay in the relationship. The abuser is often contrite, attentive, and gives the victim gifts. Both partners are in denial about the previous abuse and are convinced (sometimes repeatedly and wrongly) that this time it will be different, that the cycle will not continue and the abuse will stop. The victim may start to believe the abuse is over. However, in most cases the honeymoon phase is temporary and eventually leads to another tension-building phase as the cycle continues.

Walker asserts that after the initial abusive incident, the relationship will enter a honeymoon phase and then the cycle will start all over again. The time that each abusive relationship takes to go through these three phases can vary from days to weeks to months to even years. The original study suggests that the time to go through an entire cycle gets shorter as time goes on, creating a tighter and tighter spiral with more frequent occurrences of abuse during each subsequent cycle. The severity of abuse also tends to get more severe as time passes. Interviews with 209 female victims of abusive relationships describe this escalating severity of violence and provide support for Walker's theory.[3]

The main criticism of Walker's theory of a predictable cycle of violence is that not all abusive relationships follow the same pattern; some relationships are either abusive all the time or the abuse occurs at unpredictable intervals. Some relationships never experience a honeymoon period. In their interviews of 75 women who had left abusive relationships, Dutton and Painter found that unpredictability and intermittency of abuse were associated with the most post-relationship stress.[4] When the abuse is unpredictable (i.e., the victim does not know when it is coming, and it does not necessarily follow a predetermined pattern), the victim may be at increased risk of developing subsequent post-traumatic stress disorder (Chapter 14). Animal studies also have shown that intermittent abuse interwoven with loving treatment produces stronger bonds between the victim and the abuser.[4]

Another criticism of the cycle of violence theory is that it describes a static interaction between the abuser and the victim.[5] In reality, many relationships are constantly changing and do not follow a predetermined pattern of abuse. Walker's theory also seems to describe a predestined pattern of behavior, with little freedom of choice. At the same time, it may give abusers an excuse for their behavior as part of an inevitable cycle of actions.

Even though Walker's cycle of violence theory does not perfectly describe all abusive relationships, it can be helpful as a model to inform healthcare providers in counseling victims.

REFERENCES

1. Walker LE. *The Battered Woman*. New York, NY: Harper & Row; 1979.
2. Toohey JS. Domestic violence and rape. *Med Clin North Am.* 2008;92:1239–1252.
3. Keller J. A Guttman scale for empiric prediction of level of domestic abuse. *J Forensic Psychol Pract.* 2005;5(4):37–48.
4. Dutton DG, Painter S. The battered woman syndrome: effects of severity and intermittency of abuse. *Am J Orthopsychiatry.* 1993;63(4):614–622.
5. Dobash RE, Dobash RP. *Women, Violence and Social Change*. New York, NY: Routledge; 1992.

Chapter 4

Child Abuse

Antoinette L. Laskey, MD, MPH

INTRODUCTION

Children as victims or witnesses of family violence are increasingly recognized as a public health issue that affects millions. The highest rate of maltreatment is among infants younger than 1 year: 21.9 per 1000.[1] Data from other sources indicate that 14% of all children in the United States experience child maltreatment.[2] Perhaps more alarming is the fact that reported cases of abuse or neglect among children represent only a small number of the actual incident cases, as evidenced by multiple national studies.[3,4] It is now well established that exposure to adverse childhood experiences (ACEs) increases an individual's lifetime risk of psychiatric morbidities, such as depression, suicidality, and post-traumatic stress disorder; substance abuse, including drugs, alcohol, and tobacco; medical conditions, such as heart disease, pulmonary disease, obesity, chronic pain, excess utilization of healthcare resources; and social problems, including homelessness, interpersonal violence, and unemployment. Further, it has been clearly demonstrated that there is a strong dose-effect response to ACEs; for each additional ACE, the risk of numerous medical, psychological, and social morbidities increases.[5-10]

It is certain that *all* healthcare providers will care for either a victim or a witness of family violence at some point in their careers. The ability to recognize these patients and provide appropriate care and services is essential to the overall health and well-being of the patient both now and in the future. In this chapter, we focus on the child as a victim. It is important to remember, however, that a child who witnesses family violence is being victimized, even if a blow is never landed on that child. Children clearly suffer when they see adults in their lives abused. For the purposes of this chapter, we focus instead on child maltreatment in the forms that specifically target children as the victim.

TYPES OF ABUSE

Children may be harmed at the hands of their caregivers in a number of ways. The media is full of accounts of physical abuse, sometimes resulting in fatalities, sexual abuse, and extreme neglect. Less often we hear of seemingly bizarre cases of factitious disorder (previously known as Munchausen syndrome by proxy). Although high-profile, dramatic, or bizarre cases garner media attention, it is the more mundane but equally harmful cases that providers confront routinely. Not all physical abuse cases result in a fatality, but a child still experiences pain and sometimes permanent disability or scarring. Some children are exposed to psychological or emotional abuse, most of which is never recognized by healthcare professionals. Neglect can take many forms, from egregious failures to protect or provide (known as acts of omission) to patients who present for medical care after what appears on the surface to be "an accident." The term *accident* implies that nothing could have averted the outcome. In many cases, however, much could have been done to avert the outcome, and it is through this act of omission or commission on the part of the caregiver that harm comes to a child.

The World Health Organization defines child maltreatment as "all forms of physical and emotional ill-treatment, sexual abuse, neglect, and exploitation that results in actual or potential harm to the child's health, development, or dignity."[11]

INCIDENCE OF ABUSE

Multiple studies over the last several decades have attempted to quantify the incidence of child abuse and neglect. However, nearly every study suffers from inherent epidemiologic flaws in capturing cases that do not always present in a clear, easy-to-diagnose fashion. Two of the most important studies to be aware of are the National Child Abuse and Neglect Data System (NCANDS) and the National Incidence Studies (NIS). Both studies serve to count the number of abused children, but they approach the issue differently. NCANDS represents data that are gathered from *reported* cases of abuse from around the United States. This, by definition, means that the case was brought to the attention of local child welfare authorities. However, it has clearly been shown that not all cases are reported to child welfare authorities, despite mandated reporting laws in all 50 states.[12-15] The NIS is conducted about every 10 years as an active form of surveillance. This study is distinct from NCANDS in that it uses community sentinels to identify cases of harm, as well as risk for harm, among children in the community. This is a much broader net that allows us to understand the scope of the problem as it occurs in a population but that may not reach medical or child welfare attention.

When one considers how these studies gather data differently, it is clear that NIS would capture more cases than NCANDS and cases in NCANDS would represent more extreme examples of child maltreatment when compared with the cases in NIS. In the child abuse literature, other approaches have been taken in an attempt to quantify actual childhood exposure to violence. Direct sampling of a population has been used in a number of studies. Examples of this methodology include the CarolinaSAFE study,[3] the National Gallup Poll,[16] and the Juvenile Victimization Questionnaire.[17] These studies involved direct questioning of either parents or children to determine exposure to various forms of child maltreatment, including physical abuse, sexual abuse, and neglect. Despite the obvious risk of recall bias and social desirability bias, each of these studies showed that anonymous surveys can collect reports of harm or potential harm to children, often higher than those identified in NCANDS or NIS. The 1995 Gallup poll found that parents reported maltreatment of children in their home at a rate 10 times higher than reported rates, and CarolinaSAFE found maternal reports of physical abuse 40 times higher, and sexual abuse reports 15 times higher, than official reports.

The data clearly show that the problem of child maltreatment is widespread. Therefore, all healthcare providers should be able to recognize signs of abuse or neglect, and all providers should remain vigilant regarding the potential for family violence among their patient population.

Numerous studies demonstrate that child neglect is far more common than child physical abuse. According to the 2007 NCANDS data (the latest available), neglect makes up nearly 60% of all reported cases of maltreatment; physical abuse comprises approximately 10% of reported cases. Sexual abuse accounts for approximately 8%. The remainder includes mixed cases of abuse, psychological abuse, or other more rare forms of abuse (e.g., medical neglect, abandonment, congenital drug addiction).[1]

Although these statistics make clear that our understanding of the scope of the problem is widely variable based on data source, the numbers that do exist are staggering. Based on NCANDS data for federal fiscal year (FFY) 2007, child maltreatment fatalities were estimated at 1760. As in years past, a plurality of victims is younger than 1 year at the time of death (42.2%), and approximately a third of victims are 1–3 years. Overall, more than three-quarters of child fatalities due to maltreatment occur in children younger than 4 years. In FFY 2007, there were more than 3.5 million reports of cases of abuse or neglect, of which nearly 800,000 were substantiated as victims of maltreatment (rate: 10.6 per 1000 children). For nonfatal abuse, nearly a third of all cases occurred among children younger than 4 years.

DEMOGRAPHICS OF VICTIMS AND PERPETRATORS

It is essential that healthcare providers understand the potential for *any* child to be a victim of abuse and *any* adult care provider for a child to be a perpetrator. There is no "profile" of victim or perpetrator that can reliably be used to determine risk for a given child. Children of all races and ethnicities are at risk for maltreatment. Although there is a reported increased rate of victimization among African American children (16.7 per 1000) compared with Hispanic children (10.3 per 1000) and white children (9.1 per 1000), biases in case reporting and case finding have been demonstrated in the literature.[18–20] Child abuse in general occurs nearly equally in boys and girls.

Certain victim factors increase the risk for abuse. Younger age is a risk factor for physical abuse and neglect, and older age is a risk factor for sexual abuse.[1] Children with special healthcare needs are at an increased risk,[21] as are children who are multiples (e.g., twins, triplets).

Data on perpetrators can be more difficult to interpret because of the inherent difficulties in identifying the specific person responsible for the harm that came to the child. In some cases, more than one perpetrator may be identified. An example of this would be a case in which a stepfather is responsible for physically beating the child and the mother fails to protect the child from harm. In this case, there are two perpetrators, one of abuse, one of neglect. In other cases, no perpetrator is ever clearly identified. To the extent that we can identify them, perpetrators overwhelmingly are parents (80%). Among parental perpetrators, mothers comprise nearly 40% of perpetrators and fathers nearly 20%. The rest are mothers with fathers (or those in a father role such as stepfather or mother's boyfriend) or fathers with caregivers in mother roles. The remaining 20% are split between 10% unknown and 10% other caregivers, such as foster parents (both related and unrelated), day care providers, and non-parental legal guardians. Among all types of maltreatment, women were more likely to be perpetrators than men (57% vs 42%). This may be related to the relative number of female caregivers compared with male caregivers. Perpetrators' race closely match victim race, as would be expected given the close association between victim and perpetrator. Among children who were victims of sexual abuse, their relationship to the perpetrator was most likely to be a friend or neighbor (58%) followed by other relatives (32%) and day care providers (24%). Neglect was most often due to acts of omission or commission by a parent.[1]

Risk factors for child maltreatment among caregivers include younger age of the mother, maternal depression or substance abuse, or a single-parent household. One study found a 50 fold increased risk of death for children in households in which an unrelated adult resided.[22] Poverty is a risk factor for child maltreatment. Importantly, children in households in which domestic violence occurs are at increased risk for physical abuse.[23-27] For this reason, even if children are not in the clinical practice of a healthcare provider, identifying family violence in the home has potential impact on children in the home.

MANDATED REPORTING: ALL HEALTHCARE PROVIDERS' RESPONSIBILITY

Since the passage of the Child Abuse Prevention and Treatment Act (CAPTA) in 1974, there has been a national minimum definition of child abuse and neglect and a mandate that each state develop reporting laws to bring these cases to the notice of child welfare authorities. All 50 states, the District of Columbia, Puerto Rico, and the US territories have mandated reporting laws in place. Some states define specifically who falls under the umbrella of "mandated reporter"; other states are universal mandated reporting states, meaning that anyone (i.e., not just healthcare providers) who has concerns of abuse or neglect in a child should make a report. In all states, healthcare providers are mandated reporters. All mandated reporting laws intentionally use vague descriptors of the level of concern a reporter must have to initiate a report. Some laws say "reason to believe" or "cause to believe"; others say "suspect" that abuse or neglect has occurred. None of the mandated reporting laws require the diagnosis be made to a reasonable degree of medical certainty *to make the report*. All mandated reporter laws include good faith exemptions from civil prosecution should it ultimately be found that maltreatment was not the cause for the injuries.

Healthcare providers are often confused by the requirement to make a report in the face of Health Insurance Portability and Accountability Act (HIPAA) requirements related to disclosure of personal health information or because of concerns about doctor–patient confidentiality. It is clear that mandated reporting laws trump "privileged communications" such as doctor–patient confidentiality as well as HIPAA. In fact, specific language within HIPAA indicates that state law overrides HIPAA when "provision of state law . . . provides for the reporting of disease or injury, child abuse, birth, or death, or for the conduct of public health surveillance, investigation or intervention."[28]

It is due to the ambiguity built into the mandated reporting laws that there remains confusion among healthcare providers regarding when they need to report. Because clinical discretion is important in making the decision and healthcare providers have varying levels of knowledge and comfort with the topic, studies have shown that there is little agreement as to when a report is made based on a clinician's differential diagnosis.[29,30] Further, studies have shown, even when healthcare providers *know* what their legal mandate is, some fail to comply. Reasons given for failing to make a report to the appropriate authorities when there is concern for child maltreatment include not wanting to be involved in the legal process, uncertainty as to the diagnosis, lack of knowledge or training about how to make the diagnosis, or feeling that the "system" doesn't work.[31] Healthcare providers are only one member of a safety net for potentially abused children. Lack of certainty in the diagnosis as a barrier to reporting is a circular argument that can leave a child at significant risk. Child welfare authorities are trained to investigate and seek further medical assistance if needed to determine whether a child has been abused. An increasing number of cases of medical malpractice and medical negligence have been brought against healthcare providers who have failed to fulfill their mandated reporting role and further harm or death comes to a child as a result.

Because each state has different wording and specifics related to mandated reporting, healthcare providers are wise to clarify the law in their area as well as the specifics of how to initiate a report with the appropriate authorities.

PROFESSIONALS INVOLVED IN THE DIAGNOSIS AND MANAGEMENT OF THE POTENTIALLY ABUSED CHILD

The diagnosis of child maltreatment can be challenging. There are many injuries that can occur as the result of accidental events as well as inflicted trauma. Some medical conditions mimic findings found in abused children. Some children may be preverbal or have developmentally limited communication skills, making it difficult or impossible to obtain an accurate history from the victim. Further compounding the difficulties in diagnosis is the fact that a caregiver may not know what really happened or knows but chooses to conceal that information from the healthcare provider. Given the complicated nature of some traumas, multiple types of professionals are frequently involved in the care of these children.

In 2007, the American Board of Pediatrics approved the subspecialty status of child abuse pediatrics (CAP).[32] This sub-board of Pediatrics requires three additional years beyond pediatric residency with training that focuses on the evaluation and management of the potentially abused child. CAP fellows work closely with specialists, such as neurosurgeons, orthopedic and trauma surgeons, burn specialists, psychiatrists, ophthalmologists, radiologists, and critical care physicians, to name a few. Additionally, there is training time dedicated to working with other non-medical professionals involved in the management of the potentially abused child, such as lawyers (both defense and prosecution attorneys), child welfare agencies, law enforcement agencies, prevention agencies, and community service providers. Fellows work with death investigators and forensic pathologists in cases of fatalities, including non-abuse fatalities, such as sudden infant death syndrome (SIDS), accidental fatalities, and suicides. Training related to courtroom testimony in child welfare cases and criminal cases is an important part of the fellowship. Professionals who complete training in this area often practice at academic medical centers or in child advocacy centers. They provide expert consultation to medical colleagues as well as to non-medical professionals investigating child abuse and neglect. Child abuse pediatricians can be located through the American Academy of Pediatrics, Section on Child Abuse and Neglect, or through the National Children's Advocacy Center (NCAC).

In cases of suspected head trauma, the involvement of neurosurgeons, ophthalmologists, and critical care specialists is important in the immediate evaluation and stabilization period. Depending on the severity of the injury, involvement of rehabilitation experts, including physiatrists, physical, occupational, and speech therapists, and neurologists, may be necessary.

In cases of fractures, orthopaedic surgeons are obvious partners in care. Primary care providers should remember, however, that their role in the care of the child is often much more comprehensive than the orthopedist's role. Primary care providers should evaluate the developmental status of a child and take a comprehensive social history as well as a very detailed injury history. This information, in conjunction with information gathered from scene investigation and witness interviews by the non-medical professionals involved in the case, is essential when determining whether an injury is most likely accidental or inflicted.

In cases of alleged sexual abuse, services available vary by location, age of patient, and timing of the event in relation to the report. Many areas have established regional referral patterns to child advocacy centers. These specialized centers have expert medical providers, often child abuse pediatricians or trained nurse practitioners, along with trained forensic interviewers. For acute assault cases (i.e., those that have typically occurred in the previous 72–96 hours, depending on the circumstances), many hospital emergency departments have sexual assault nurse examiners to aid in forensic evidence collection and injury documentation. It should be noted that, when possible, it is best practice to assure that the provider of these acute sexual assault evaluations is adequately trained in the unique circumstances and evaluation techniques used in pre-adolescent patients. Adult sexual assault evaluation practices are not all applicable or appropriate for children or young adolescents. Forensic interviewers may be social workers or law enforcement agents. Unless there are no medical providers in the environment who are trained in such reporting, rarely should an untrained healthcare provider take a detailed sexual assault or sexual abuse history. Histories can be contaminated through improper questions or phrases. Medical history-taking, especially when related to the body systems involved, is the purview of the healthcare provider and should be part of a complete evaluation.

Abusive injuries that result in cutaneous findings, such as burns, bruises, cuts, pattern injuries (e.g., belt marks, loop marks, hand prints), or scars may require the assistance of burn surgeons, often plastic surgeons, dermatologists, rheumatologists, infectious disease experts, or a general pediatrician with a broad knowledge base of skin findings in pediatrics. Oral injuries may require dental specialties including oral maxillofacial surgeons or otolaryngologists and dentists. Overall, it is important to remember when evaluating a child for potential inflicted injuries that collaboration with medical specialists is imperative.

Just as collaboration with medical colleagues is critical in the provision of quality care, so is the importance of recognizing the limitations of healthcare providers in evaluating risks to a patient based on our typically time-limited interactions with a family. Seeing a patient for small snapshots in time makes us rely on other professionals to fully assess the safety of a child. This becomes an issue when healthcare providers note the "obvious concern" of a caregiver or the "lack of fear" of a child toward a caregiver. Although this may in fact be the case, healthcare providers are often not privy to the child's actual living conditions or typically do not have access to all of the care providers in the child's life. This is where the non-medical professionals involved in child protection are so important. Child welfare agencies serve a vital role in protecting children; their involvement does not guarantee a child will be removed from their home. Many states have provisions that if, after an investigation, it is found that additional support services would benefit a child and family, rather than outright removal, those services can be offered (and in some cases mandated). Further, through professional investigations, additional information may be discovered that clarifies the circumstances surrounding an injury, permitting determination that the injury was due to an accident rather than abuse, for instance.

In addition to child welfare agencies, law enforcement may assist in an investigation, depending on the state and locale in which an event occurs.

Frequently, these agencies work together on an investigation. As mentioned earlier, HIPAA does not prevent a healthcare provider from discussing a case of child abuse with the appropriate authorities conducting an investigation. Guardian *ad litems* (GALs) or court-appointed special advocates (CASAs) may be professionals or lay individuals with training in child abuse and neglect cases appointed by the courts to represent a child through the legal and social service system. They literally are assigned to be the voice for the child. Commonly, GALs or CASAs contact healthcare providers involved in a child's care with questions related to ongoing treatment issues, findings, or medical questions related to the child's conditions. Because they are appointed by the courts to represent the child, they have official documentation identifying their role in the child's care.

GENERAL MANAGEMENT ISSUES

As with any medical condition, the ABCs are paramount. All providers must first assure that airway-breathing-circulation is stable before moving on with the assessment. Similarly, as with most medical conditions, the history is key to identifying and understanding the problem at hand. In cases that may involve child abuse and neglect, accurate history-taking is vital. Open-ended questions should be asked whenever possible. Obtaining specific details is also important. For example, when evaluating a child with a fracture, it is not enough to know there is a reported fall; it is important to document how the fall occurred, the estimated distance, the surface contacted, the body surface that hit, and so on. One also should know about the child's developmental capabilities. Although young infants cannot roll over on their own, if placed in certain positions on certain surfaces, they may be able to squirm their way off or kick themselves off. This is where developmental history and detailed injury event history can be illustrative. Using the exact words or phrases reported is helpful to avoid the proverbial game of "telephone." This happens when each medical provider paraphrases various parts of a history and, as the history is repeated over time, changes occur, sometimes resulting in the caregiver being accused of a "changing history" that can be concerning for abuse.

 If children are verbal, it is appropriate to ask in a non-leading way why they believe that they are seeing the doctor. It should be kept in mind that if there is concern the caregiver present may be responsible for the injuries or events that led to presentation to medical care, it is not appropriate to question the child in front of this caregiver. Asking the child to report what happened is appropriate; it is *not* appropriate to ask leading questions like, "Did your mommy hurt you?", "Did your daddy touch your private area?", or other questions that presume an event. It is better to ask questions such as, "Can you tell me why you are here today?" Any spontaneous disclosures made by a child should be documented clearly, using quotes and the exact words, not paraphrasing. One should not assume that when a child identifies a caregiver as "Dad" or "Mom" that the person is actually the father or mother. It may be a name used for more than one male or female in the child's life. A complete social history is imperative for understanding the social milieu of the family. Additionally, a thorough family history is necessary to direct further testing, as necessary, related to conditions such as inherited bleeding disorders or bone pathology.

After the history is taken, a complete and thorough physical examination should be obtained. It is rarely sufficient to examine a child with clothes on. Important findings may be identified only through a complete skin exam. Head circumferences in children younger than three years should be documented and plotted on growth charts. A head that is too big for chronological age may indicate an underlying pathology. Complete physical exams include examination of the genitals. Often physicians feel uncomfortable doing this and miss important information about the health of the child. Determining the Tanner stage of the child is important for developmental reasons. Examining the genitals may reveal medical pathology unrelated to abuse but important nonetheless. It is common for clinicians to not feel comfortable examining the female child's genitalia because little attention is given to the normal anatomy during medical school or residency. It should be noted that the hymen *must* have an opening in it from birth. This is not a sign of penetration; it is anatomically normal. In fact, the absence of a hole in the hymen is distinctly abnormal and requires medical intervention for imperforate hymen.

Any injuries identified during the examination should be clearly documented, in detail with measurements when possible. Photos are useful to further describe findings. Digital photography is acceptable and may be used as evidence in legal proceedings. When photographing injuries, the following should be included in the photo: patient identifiers, a size standard (e.g., a ruler when possible; a coin is acceptable if no ruler is available), and close-up and overall pictures of the area. There should be documentation in the medical record that photos were taken and where those photos can be found if not in the actual chart. Sometimes injuries need to be followed and documented over time. This is the case especially for slap marks, bite marks, and other injuries that may evolve over time. There is no scientific foundation for dating of bruises by visual inspection. Multiple research studies have shown variations in color perception limit between-observer reliability in assigning a color to a bruise and that color evolution depends on many individual characteristics, such as hematocrit, body fat, skin complexion, and location of the bruise. It is never appropriate to speculate on the age of a bruise.[33–36]

Accurate documentation is important in any medical record. However, in cases of potential child maltreatment, excellent documentation is paramount. There are multiple professionals who will rely on the history and the physical exam findings recorded in the medical record. If this information is cursory, illegible, or indecipherable for any reason (e.g., because of idiomatic jargon or abbreviations), the information contained is not useful. Care should be taken to document everything as clearly, accurately, and objectively as possible. Although there is a role for a medical professional to offer his or her subjective assessment of the situation, it is not helpful to have subjective assessments throughout the record. Examples of this are when providers posit opinions such as "The mother could not have caused these injuries as she clearly loves the child" or "The child exhibits no fear of his caregiver; therefore I have no concerns about abuse." Clear, precise documentation is essential to enhance the communication among the various professionals involved in the care of these children.

After the physical examination is complete, a further medical workup may be needed. Radiology and blood studies are the most common examples. For children 2 years or younger who are being evaluated for physical abuse, it is mandatory that a complete skeletal survey be done[37,38] (Table 4–1). In children 2–5 years, clinical discretion dictates when a skeletal survey is completed. Skeletal surveys are rarely clinically appropriate in children older than 5 years. Important findings identified on skeletal surveys include rib fractures, metaphyseal corner fractures, or occult fractures with evidence of healing. It is unusual that fractures in young children have bruising and/or swelling associated with them. It is not appropriate to screen for fractures using just a physical examination in infants and young children.

Table 4–1 Minimum Skeletal Survey Requirements

- Humeri (AP)
- Forearms (AP)
- Hands (PA)
- Femurs (AP)
- Lower legs (AP)
- Feet (PA or AP)
- Thorax: ribs, thoracic spine, and upper lumbar spine (AP and lateral)
- Pelvis and mid lumbar spine (AP)
- Lumbosacral spine (lateral)
- Cervical spine (AP and lateral)
- Skull (frontal and lateral)
- Optional: oblique rib views

AP, anteroposterior; L, lumbar; PA, posteroanterior; T, thoracic.

In children younger than 2 years, it is also imperative to consider the possibility of occult intracranial injury. Studies have shown that intracranial injuries may be missed by healthcare providers or be clinically silent at presentation for other injuries.[18,39,40] Cranial imaging, therefore, is warranted in the evaluation of physical abuse in young children. Head computed tomography (CT) using as low as reasonably achievable (ALARA) protocols for children or magnetic resonance imaging (MRI) where available are important adjuncts to the evaluation.

Blood work should not be ordered without considering its purpose. If the presenting findings are manifested by bruising or bleeding (as in cases of intracranial hemorrhage), bleeding evaluations are appropriate. This would include complete blood counts and coagulation panels.[41] Depending on the findings on physical exam and the lab results, further testing might be warranted, such as factor analyses or platelet function tests, or guided by consultation with a pediatric hematologist. If the evaluation reveals fractures, basic chemistries, including magnesium, calcium, phosphorous, and alkaline phosphatase, should be considered. In some cases, vitamin D studies are indicated, especially if the child might be at particular risk for rickets.[42] In cases of physical abuse, occult abdominal trauma should be considered. Liver function tests, especially elevations of aspartate aminotransferase and alanine aminotransferase, are useful for identifying occult abdominal injury.[43] Some conditions, such as osteogenesis imperfecta, can mimic non-accidental/inflicted injury and require collaboration with genetic specialists.

If a child is being evaluated for an acute sexual assault, several laboratory tests are indicated. Currently, the use of urine tests, such as nucleic acid amplification tests for gonorrhea and chlamydia, are not approved for use in pre-pubescent children. Therefore, when testing for sexually transmitted infections, cultures should be used. Chlamydia, gonorrhea, syphilis (STIs), and human immunodeficiency virus (HIV) acquired outside of the perinatal period are considered diagnostic of child sexual abuse. Herpes simplex and human papillomavirus can be transmitted sexually or through non-sexual contact. Consultation with a child abuse pediatrician is recommended if there are concerns about sexually transmitted infections in pre-adolescent children. Blood tests for syphilis, HIV, and hepatitis B and C should be considered based on the reported type of contact and risk factors in the alleged perpetrator. As post-sexual assault prophylaxis changes due to resistance patterns in the community, it is important that clinicians consult the Centers for Disease Control and Prevention (CDC) Web site to determine the currently appropriate treatment regimen. If the patient is an adolescent girl, pregnancy testing is imperative. Pap smears are not considered part of the routine evaluation related to a sexual assault.

Aside from the medical management of the patient, the child welfare component needs to be addressed. When the evaluation has progressed to the point that the provider feels there is "cause to believe" that the child is a victim of abuse, a report to the appropriate authorities should be made. Information about the injuries found, history given, and caregivers for the child should be provided to child welfare. It is also important to notify child welfare if there are other children in the same environment as the patient when the events may have occurred. This is information that needs to be conveyed in a timely fashion because these children may also be in harm's way. The circumstances of a given case will dictate the evaluation that should be pursued for other children exposed to the same environment or caregivers.

Follow-up after discharge from care for the acute injuries is vital to the ongoing well-being of the child. Some injuries require extensive follow-up care and subspecialty evaluations. Other children require ongoing psychological follow-up and support. For a primary healthcare provider, care coordination is an important duty.

OUTCOMES

Not surprisingly, the long- and short-term outcomes resulting from child maltreatment are wide ranging. Death in the immediate time surrounding the abusive event may occur. There is the obvious short-term morbidity associated with any inflicted injury, whether from physical or sexual abuse. Studies show that the morbidity associated with inflicted traumatic brain injuries when compared with accidental head injuries is more significant with higher injury severity scores, longer stays in intensive care, and higher per-hospitalization expenditure.[44] Delays in care can often result in increased morbidity, as can be seen in burns (increased infection, increased scarring) or in inflicted head injuries (worse outcomes due to secondary brain injuries).

Long-term outcomes vary by type of maltreatment. Survivors of severe inflicted traumatic brain injuries often die at an early age as a direct result of their brain damage. Outcomes that include seizures, paralysis, blindness, or deafness are not uncommon. It is estimated that approximately a third of abusive head injuries result in death in the immediate post-event period, a third lead to permanent disability or impairment, and a third will appear relatively normal at discharge. Of this final third, however, it is known that the true outcome cannot be determined until these children reach school age. Long-term follow-up of these survivors shows that they often go on to have difficulty with learning or behavior when they enter the structured school environment. It also has been shown that the lifetime cost to provide care to survivors of abusive head trauma can run into the millions of dollars.

In cases of sexual abuse and sexual assault, providers need to remain attuned to the possibility of psychological morbidity. Crisis counseling immediately after the event(s) is disclosed is important for dealing with the psychological crises both the victim and the family may experience. However, it is not unusual that ongoing or intermittent counseling also is warranted. Referring a child and his or her family as needed to appropriate counseling resources is an important role of the primary care provider. The age and developmental level of the child should be considered, as well as the counselor's or psychologist's ability to deal specifically with this topic.

As mentioned earlier, adverse childhood experiences can lead directly to impairments in an adult's life. Primary care providers for adult patients should be aware that unresolved traumatic childhood issues can continue to cause problems in all areas of an adult's life.[5,45]

CONCLUSION

Child maltreatment affects millions of children in the United States each year, costing billions of dollars to treat immediate and long-term consequences, and results in harm that is both immediate and long lasting. Prevention efforts are crucial to deal with what is clearly a public health crisis. Prevention can take many forms and can be offered at both the family and societal levels. As science evolves and we understand more about the types of harm children may suffer at the hands of their caregivers, we need to work even harder to develop effective prevention strategies. Stopping the cycle of family violence is crucial to the future of our children.

REFERENCES

1. U.S. Department of Health and Human Services Administration on Children, Youth and Families. *Child Maltreatment 2007.* Washington, DC: USDHHS; 2009.
2. Finkelhor D, Ormrod R, Turner H, et al. The victimization of children and youth: a comprehensive, national survey [published correction appears in *Child Maltreat.* 2005;10(2):207]. *Child Maltreat.* 2005;10(1):5–25.
3. Theodore AD, Chang JJ, Runyan DK, Hunter WM, Bangdiwala SI, Agans R. Epidemiologic features of the physical and sexual maltreatment of children in the Carolinas. *Pediatrics.* 2005;115(3):e331–337.
4. U.S. Department of Health and Human Services. *Third National Incidence Study of Child Abuse and Neglect.* Washington, DC: USDHHS; 1996.

5. Anda RF, Felitti VJ, Bremner JD, et al. The enduring effects of abuse and related adverse experiences in childhood. A convergence of evidence from neurobiology and epidemiology. *Eur Arch Psychiatry Clin Neurosci.* 2006;256(3):174–186.

6. Dube SR, Anda RF, Felitti VJ, Chapman DP, Williamson DF, Giles WH. Childhood abuse, household dysfunction, and the risk of attempted suicide throughout the life span: findings from the Adverse Childhood Experiences Study. *JAMA.* 2001;286(24):3089–3096.

7. Dube SR, Anda RF, Whitfield CL, et al. Long-term consequences of childhood sexual abuse by gender of victim. *Am J Prevent Med.* 2005;28(5):430–438.

8. Felitti VJ, Anda RF, Nordenberg D, et al. Relationship of childhood abuse and household dysfunction to many of the leading causes of death in adults. The Adverse Childhood Experiences (ACE) Study. *Am J Prevent Med.* 1998;14(4):245–258.

9. Hillis SD, Anda RF, Felitti VJ, Marchbanks PA. Adverse childhood experiences and sexual risk behaviors in women: a retrospective cohort study. *Fam Plann Perspect.* 2001;33(5):206–211.

10. Hillis SD, Anda RF, Felitti VJ, Nordenberg D, Marchbanks PA. Adverse childhood experiences and sexually transmitted diseases in men and women: a retrospective study. *Pediatrics.* 2000;106(1):E11.

11. Child maltreatment. World Health Organization Web site. http://www. who.int/topics/child_abuse/en/. Accessed January 2010.

12. Flaherty E, Sege R, Dhepyasuwan N, Price LL, Wasserman R. Child abuse (CA) suspicion and reporting among primary care practitioners (PCPs). Paper presented at: Pediatric Academic Society Meeting, May 17, 2005; Washington, DC.

13. Flaherty EG, Sege R, Price LL, Christoffel KK, Norton DP, O'Connor KG. Pediatrician characteristics associated with child abuse identification and reporting: results from a national survey of pediatricians. *Child Maltreat.* 2006;11(4):361–369.

14. Flaherty EG, Sege RD, Griffith J, et al. From suspicion of physical child abuse to reporting: primary care clinician decision-making. *Pediatrics.* 2008;122(3): 611–619.

15. Jones R, Flaherty EG, Binns HJ, et al. Clinicians' description of factors influencing their reporting of suspected child abuse: report of the Child Abuse Reporting Experience Study Research Group. *Pediatrics.* 2008;122(2): 259–266.

16. Gallup G, Gallup J. *The Gallup Poll: Public Opinion 1995.* Lanham, MD: SR Books; 1995.

17. Finkelhor D, Hamby SL, Ormrod R, et al. The Juvenile Victimization Questionnaire: reliability, validity, and national norms. *Child Abuse Negl.* 2005;29(4):383–412.

18. Jenny C, Hymel KP, Ritzen A, Reinert SE, Hay TC. Analysis of missed cases of abusive head trauma. *JAMA.* 1999;281(7):621–626.

19. Hampton RL, Newberger EH. Child abuse incidence and reporting by hospitals: significance of severity, class, and race. *Am J Public Health.* 1985;75(1):56–60.

20. Lane WG, Rubin DM, Monteith R, Christian CW. Racial differences in the evaluation of pediatric fractures for physical abuse. *JAMA.* 2002;288(13):1603–1609.

21. Hibbard RA, Desch LW. Maltreatment of children with disabilities. *Pediatrics.* 2007;119(5):1018–1025.

22. Schnitzer PG, Ewigman BG. Child deaths resulting from inflicted injuries: household risk factors and perpetrator characteristics. *Pediatrics.* 2005;116(5):e687–693.

23. Coohey C, Braun N. Toward an integrated framework for understanding child physical abuse. *Child Abuse Negl.* 1997;21(11):1081–1094.

24. McGuigan WM, Pratt CC. The predictive impact of domestic violence on three types of child maltreatment. *Child Abuse Negl.* 2001;25(7):869–883.

25. Rumm PD, Cummings P, Krauss MR, Bell MA, Rivara FP. Identified spouse abuse as a risk factor for child abuse. *Child Abuse Negl.* 2000;24(11):1375–1381.

26. Herrenkohl TI, Sousa C, Tajima EA, et al. Intersection of child abuse and children's exposure to domestic violence. *Trauma, Violence Abuse.* 2008;9(2):84–99.

27. Tajima EA. The relative importance of wife abuse as a risk factor for violence against children. *Child Abuse Negl.* 2000;24(11):1383–1398.

28. Committee on Child Abuse and Neglect. Child abuse, confidentiality, and the Health Insurance Portability and Accountability Act. *Pediatrics.*125(1):197–201.

29. Levi BH, Brown G. Reasonable suspicion: a study of Pennsylvania pediatricians regarding child abuse. *Pediatrics.* 2005;116(1):e5–12.

30. Levi BH, Brown G, Erb C. Reasonable suspicion: a pilot study of pediatric residents. *Child Abuse Negl.* 2006;30(4):345–356.

31. Flaherty EG, Sege R, Binns HJ, Mattson CL, Christoffel KK. Health care providers' experience reporting child abuse in the primary care setting. Pediatric Practice Research Group. *Arch Pediatr Adolesc Med.* 2000;154(5):489–493.

32. Block RW, Palusci VJ. Child abuse pediatrics: a new pediatric subspecialty. *J Pediatr.* 2006;148(6):711–712.

33. Bariciak ED, Plint AC, Gaboury I, Bennett S. Dating of bruises in children: an assessment of physician accuracy. *Pediatrics.* 2003;112(4):804–807.

34. Maguire S, Mann MK, Sibert J, Kemp A. Can you age bruises accurately in children? A systematic review. *Arch Dis Child.* 2005;90(2):187–189.

35. Munang LA, Leonard PA, Mok JY. Lack of agreement on colour description between clinicians examining childhood bruising. *J Clin Forensic Med.* 2002;9(4):171–174.

36. Stephenson T, Bialas Y. Estimation of the age of bruising. *Arch Dis Child.* 1996;74(1):53–55.

37. Diagnostic imaging of child abuse. *Pediatrics.* 2009;123(5):1430–1435.

38. American College of Radiology. ACR practice guideline for skeletal surveys in children. 2006. Available at http://www.acr.org/secondarymainmenucategories/ quality_safety/guidelines/pediatric/skeletal_surveys.aspx. Accessed January 15, 2010.

39. Rubin DM, Christian CW, Bilaniuk LT, Zazyczny KA, Durbin DR. Occult head injury in high-risk abused children. *Pediatrics.* 2003;111(6 Pt 1):1382–1386.

40. Laskey AL, Holsti M, Runyan DK, Socolar RR. Occult head trauma in young suspected victims of physical abuse. *J Pediatr.* 2004;144(6):719–722.

41. Acosta M, Edwards R, Jaffe EI, Yee DL, Mahoney DH, Teruya J. A practical approach to pediatric patients referred with an abnormal coagulation profile. *Arch Pathol Lab Med.* 2005;129(8):1011–1016.

42. Misra M, Pacaud D, Petryk A, Collett-Solberg PF, Kappy M. Vitamin D deficiency in children and its management: review of current knowledge and recommendations. *Pediatrics.* 2008;122(2):398–417.

43. Lindberg D, Makoroff K, Harper N, et al. Utility of hepatic transaminases to recognize abuse in children. *Pediatrics*. 2009;124(2):509–516.
44. Ettaro L, Berger RP, Songer T. Abusive head trauma in young children: characteristics and medical charges in a hospitalized population. *Child Abuse Negl*. 2004;28(10):1099–1111.
45. Felitti VJ. The relationship of adverse childhood experiences to adult medical disease, psychiatric disorders, and sexual behavior: implications for healthcare. In: Lanius R, Vermetten, Pain C, eds. *The Hidden Epidemic: The Impact of Early Life Trauma on Health and Disease*. Atlanta, GA: Cambridge University Press; 2009.

Chapter 5

Bullying

Sarina Schrager, MD, MS

INTRODUCTION

Bullying is defined as the use of aggression to cause harm to another person.[1] The bully (or the person who exhibits bullying behavior) has power, and the victim (or the person who is in the victim role) does not. Bullying implies repeated acts of aggression, usually happening at school where the person doing the bullying continues the behavior in spite of the obvious distress of the victim. Bullying can be further classified as physical aggression and psychological or emotional aggression (e.g., name-calling, exclusion from groups). Bullying also occurs on the Internet. So-called cyber-bullying can have a profound impact on a young person's life. Children who bully are more likely to carry weapons to school and to be involved in physical fights.[1] Both bullies and victims of bullying can demonstrate long-lasting physical and psychological effects related to the bullying.

CHARACTERISTICS OF CHILDREN INVOLVED IN BULLYING

Multiple children can be involved in the bullying—not just the children who bully and those who are victims. Bullying does not usually happen in a vacuum. Other children are often aware of the bullying behavior. Children can assist the bully, support the bullying behavior by encouraging the bully, or pretend they do not know about the bullying.[1] Children also can help defend the victim by confronting the bully or telling a teacher or principal.[1]

Bullying can be a one-on-one interaction, or a group of children can bully one victim or a group of victims. In many cases, teachers and other adults have some sense that the bullying is occurring, but often do not intervene spontaneously. Bullying can occur anywhere, but school (e.g., on the play-ground at recess, in the hallways, in the cafeteria) or on the way to and from school are the most common places.[1] Children who are overweight or have physical disabilities are at higher risk of being bullied, as are children who are homosexual or transgendered.[1] Children new to a school may also be at higher risk of bullying because of a lack of friends or other social support networks.

DEMOGRAPHICS

Bullying is common. Evaluation of the 2005 Health Behavior in School Age Children survey that included more than 7000 nationally representative 6th to 10th graders showed that children's experience of bullying within the previous 2 months was very high.[2] In this cohort, more than 20% of the children reported physical bullying, 53% reported verbal bullying, 51% reported social bullying, and 13% reported electronic or Internet bullying.[2] This cohort demonstrated that boys were more likely to be involved in physical or verbal bullying, whereas girls were more likely to be involved in social bullying (e.g., excluding others from their social group).[2] A US Department of Education study from 2007 found that 32% of children between 12 and 18 years described being bullied during the previous year.[3] Almost 23% of girls in this study described being subjects of rumors compared with 13.5% of boys.[3] Bullying became less common as the children aged, ranging from more than 42% of 6th graders to 23% of 12th graders.[3] Bullying in elementary schools is less common, with one study finding that 19% of elementary school children in the United States were bullied.[4] Children who are bullied frequently have chronic nonspecific physical symptoms, including headaches, difficulty sleeping, abdominal pain, anxiety and/or depression, alcohol or substance abuse, and lower school achievement.[5] Children who bully may show similar physical and psychological symptoms. Parents also may notice that children who bully may not show concern for other people's feelings and also may bully younger siblings.[5] The longer that the bullying behavior occurs, and the more severe it is, the more likely that the children involved in it will develop these associated problems.[5]

Cyber-bullying is becoming more common. Several cases of cyber-bullying leading to suicide have been reported in the popular press and underline the seriousness of this issue. Cyber-bullying is the act of using electronic media (e.g., the Internet, texting, Twitter, and Facebook) to spread rumors, gossip, or misinformation about others. The estimate of the incidence of cyber-bullying ranges from 23% to 72% among middle and high school students.[6] Cyber-bullying is more public than individual bullying and may also be performed by adults. With the advent of social media (i.e., Facebook and Twitter), gossip and name-calling can be disseminated to tens or hundreds or even thousands of recipients within minutes. The risks of cyber-bullying are related to typical bullying behavior (i.e., children who bully regularly are more likely to be involved in cyber-bullying) and amount of time spent on the Internet (the more time online, the greater the risk of cyber-bullying).[6] Most victims of cyber-bullying know the perpetrators.[6]

PREDICTORS OF BULLYING

Children who bully do have some common personality characteristics. They are more likely to be impulsive, have a positive attitude toward violence, and have trouble following rules.[1] Many children who bully do not have involved parents, but some do. Children who bully are at greater future risk of violence, drug and alcohol use, and, in boys, criminal convictions as adults.[1] Children who bully should be screened for conduct disorder and other psychiatric comorbidities.[1] Children who are bullied have fewer sequelae if they have involved and caring adults in their lives, are trained in social skills and negotiation, and a have strong social support system.[1] Both children who bully and those who are bullied are more likely to do poorly in school or drop out of school.[5]

Exposure to family violence (FV) (either as direct child abuse—physical or verbal—or as a witness to parental intimate partner violence [IPV]) may be a risk factor for bullying among children. A cross-sectional study of more than a thousand Italian elementary and middle school children found that exposure to IPV in their homes was directly correlated to the risk of bullying or victimization at school.[7] One study of 5- to 7-year-olds also found that exposure to IPV at home was a risk factor for bullying;[8] another smaller study of 112 6- to 13-year-olds did not.[9] However, despite the lack of direct association found in the second study, children who witnessed IPV demonstrated more physical aggressive behaviors.[9]

Sexual bullying may be a particular issue for adolescents. Some theories identify sexual bullying (e.g., pressuring someone to have sexual intercourse or to perform sexual acts they do not want to do, or receiving unwanted sexual attention) as a new concept that links childhood bullying to dating violence or sexual assault.[10] Sexual bullying is most common in middle school or young high school students when adolescents start to have relationships but are not really dating yet.

SCREENING

Because of the high prevalence of bullying and the associated conditions, clinicians may want to screen high-risk children for bullying behavior. Four questions that can help identify children who bully or are bullied include (1) "How often does the bullying behavior happen?", (2) "How long has it been going on?", (3) "Where does the bullying occur?", and (4) "What actually happens during the bullying and how does it make you feel?"[5] Bullying that occurs more frequently, has lasted a long time, and occurs in more than one venue puts the child at highest risk for developing chronic physical and psychological issues (as described earlier).[11]

PREVENTION

Most prevention programs occur at school.[12] Schools have tried curriculum prevention programs, in which the students hear didactic presentations about bullying and/or participate in social skills groups. Some schools have hired more social workers to help the students. Others have developed programs that include many individual students and classrooms.[12] Prevention of bullying is most successful when it is multidimensional.[12] The programs that seem to have worked best involve a combination of new school rules, teacher training, student curriculum, training about conflict resolution, and individual counseling.[12] One of the most effective programs for reduction of bullying among elementary and middle school students is the Olweus Bullying Prevention program, which was developed in Norway.[13] This program sets schoolwide standards that do not tolerate bullying, provides support for victims, and tries to change the culture that has traditionally tolerated bullying.[13]

CONCLUSION

Bullying is an important issue that clinicians, teachers, parents, and society in general must identify to prevent further school violence and adolescent suicide. Clinicians should have a high level of suspicion for bullying in children with chronic nonspecific physical or psychological complaints, change in school performance, or new use of tobacco, drugs, or alcohol.

REFERENCES

1. Lyznicki JM, McCaffree MA, Robinowitz CR. Childhood bullying: implications for physicians. *Am Fam Physician.* 2004;70(9):1723–1728, 1729–1730.
2. Wang J, Iannotti RJ, Nansel TR. School bullying among adolescents in the United States: physical, verbal, relational, and cyber. *J Adolesc Health.* 2009;45(4):368–375.

3. Indicators of school crime and safety: 2009. National Center for Education Statistics Web site. http://nces.ed.gov/programs/crimeindicators/crimeindicators2009/tables/table_11_1.asp?referrer=report. Accessed April 25, 2010.

4. Dake JA, Price JH, Telljohann SK. The nature and extent of bullying at school. *J School Health.* 2003;73(5):173–180.

5. Lamb J, Pepler DJ, Craig W. Approach to bullying and victimization. *Can Fam Physician.* 2009;55:356–360.

6. Guan SSA, Subrahmanyam K. Youth Internet use: risks and opportunities. *Cur Opin Psychol.* 2009;22:351–356.

7. Baldry AC. Bullying in schools and exposure to domestic violence. *Child Abuse Negl.* 2003;27:713–732.

8. Bowes L, Arseneault L, Maughan B, Taylor A, Caspi A, Moffit TE. School, neighborhood, and family factors are associated with children's bullying involvement: a nationally representative longitudinal study. *J Am Acad Child Adolesc Psychol.* 2009;48(5):545–553.

9. Bauer NS, Herrenkohl TI, Lozano P, Rivara FP, Hill KG, Hawkins JD. Childhood bullying involvement and exposure to intimate partner violence. *Pediatrics.* 2006;118(2):e235-242.

10. Fredland NM. Sexual bullying: addressing the gap between bullying and dating violence. *Adv Nurs Sci.* 2008;31(2):95–105.

11. Craig WM, Pepler DJ. Identifying and targeting risk for involvement in bullying and victimization. *Can J Psychiatry.* 2003;48(9):577–582.

12. Vreeman RC, Carroll AE. A systematic review of school-based interventions to prevent bullying. *Arch Pediatr Adolesc Med.* 2007;161:78–88.

13. Olweus D. *Bullying at School: What We Know and What We Can Do.* Cambridge, MA: Blackwell; 1993.

Chapter 6

Intimate Partner Violence

DaWana Stubbs, MD, MS
Rose S. Fife, MD, MPH

INTRODUCTION

Intimate partner violence (IPV) is a public health epidemic affecting people of all ages, races/ethnicities, religions, and socioeconomic levels. Although both genders can be victims of IPV, 85% of IPV involves women being abused by men.[1] Women at the greatest risk for experiencing abuse are those who are unmarried, younger than 35 years, and have an annual income below $15,000.[2,3] However, data have shown that anyone, no matter what a person's racial/ethnic or socioeconomic status, can be a victim.[4] It has been estimated that almost 5 million women in the United States are physically assaulted each year by intimate partners.[5] Approximately 17,000 homicides are due to IPV each year in the United States, and most of the victims are women.[1,5] Almost a third of female victims of homicide are killed by intimate partners.[1,5] Abused women are at increased risk of problems with pregnancy and childbirth, depression and anxiety, substance abuse, and chronic medical illnesses.[5-7]

Abused women use health care at higher rates than their non-abused counterparts.[8,9,10] Medical and mental health costs for IPV injuries are more than $4 million annually.[1] IPV results in the loss of approximately 8 million days of work a year.[1]

RECOGNITION

IPV can occur in several forms, including emotional, verbal, financial, sexual, and physical abuse. Emotional abuse can include trickery, dishonesty, lying to others about the victim, and jealousy. Verbal abuse can include yelling, insults, derogatory comments, and sexual comments. Financial abuse may include making victims ask for money and preventing them from getting or keeping a job or from keeping the money she or he earns. Sexual abuse can be the most difficult for women to discuss and may include rape, unwanted sexual contact, rude comments, and not listening to "no." The most notable form is physical abuse, which usually escalates in both frequency and severity and may be fatal. Physical abuse includes a wide range of actions, including destroying property, blocking one's path, spitting, slapping, pulling hair, pushing, punching, kicking, choking, throwing things, using weapons, punching walls, and breaking things in sight of the other person. Being the target of such acts can produce feelings of helplessness, worthlessness, shame, and depression.[11-13]

The common physical injuries and medical findings suggestive of abuse include, but are not limited to, the following:

- Somatic disorders
- Depression
- Anxiety
- Chronic pain syndromes
- Story and injury inconsistencies
- Injuries to face, torso, breast, abdomen (central distribution)
- Defensive injuries to the forearms
- Injuries/bruises in different stages of healing
- Any type of injury caused by sexual assault
- Delay in seeking treatment
- Gynecologic complications, such as miscarriages, premature rupture of membranes, abruptio placentae, antepartum hemorrhage (see Chapter 7)

DOCUMENTATION

The most important part of screening and documentation is to maintain the patient's confidentially. Any discussion of IPV should be conducted in private. The partner or anyone else close to the patient should not be present during the screening process.[14-16]

Framing statements should be used to open the discussion of IPV. These statements help to destigmatize the issue and produce a feeling of not being singled out. For example, "I ask all of my patients about their relationships and family so I can understand them better and be available to discuss any problems they may be experiencing."[14]

Once the door has been opened, and depending on the initial discussion, providers can ask either indirect or direct questions. Indirect questions remain fairly general but allow for a deeper inquiry into possible abuse. An example may be: "Every couple fights. What are fights or disagreements like in your home? Do they ever become physical?" Direct questions should be used if indirect questioning, physical examination, or other observation raises any suspicion of current abuse. For example, such questions might include "Has your partner or ex-partner ever hit or hurt you?" or "Has your partner or ex-partner ever threatened to hurt you or someone close to you?"[14] Studies show that abused women prefer and appreciate their physician asking direct questions[16] and openly discuss any clinical suspicion of abuse.[17] Many consider this a better way to approach the problem than to expect a woman to volunteer such information spontaneously.[16] IPV is associated with significant stigma in most groups, and women (and especially men) are usually unwilling to initiate the conversation spontaneously with the healthcare provider.[11-13] Ancillary staff in the provider's office also may start the conversation, and, in some cases, the victim may feel more comfortable with such assistants than they do with physicians. An office nurse or medical assistant, especially one who is a woman and one with whom the victim may better identify, can serve as a good conduit for the initial discussion and for episodic follow-up. In some offices, such staff are trained in directing the victim to resources available in the community to help her. However, the primary provider must remain engaged in the discussions throughout (see Chapter 17).

If screening reveals abuse, it should be documented like any other medical problem. Good documentation is usually very helpful to the patient in both criminal and civil court proceedings. Documentation can occur in three forms: as a written description, freehand or printed sketches, and photos.[18]

The written description should be framed in neutral and nonjudgmental language that outlines the chronology of the event(s) in the patient's words and describes the physical findings.[14] The healthcare provider should avoid phrases or words that sound either belittling or blaming and give the impression of disbelief, such as: *"Is that all?," "just claims," and "only."*[19] The written description should include answers to the following questions:

- Who injured you?
- How is the batterer related to you?
- How many times has this happened before?
- When was the last episode? What is the worst episode you can remember?
- Were any children at home during the abuse? If so, were they injured?[1]

Freehand or printed sketches can be used as an adjunct to the written narrative. The provider should record all new or old injuries, showing their location, size, depth, and appearance.[18] Any areas that the patient reports as being tender should be noted because bruising may appear later. Any photos of injuries should be documented and linked to the sketch. Photographs provide additional information and should be obtained only with the patient's consent. Photographs should be taken with color film, using either a ruler or other standardized object in the photo to clarify the size of the wound or bruise. Photos should be taken from different angles before medical treatment is given, and at least one should include the patient's face. All photos should be labeled with the name of the patient and photographer, location of the injury, and the date.[18]

HEALTH CONSEQUENCES

The physical and mental sequelae of IPV have been well documented[6–9] and can have an effect long after the abuse has ended[6,7] with symptom severity increasing with duration of the abuse.[8,9,20] Both psychological and physical abuse are associated with poor health outcomes.[9] Women who have experienced abuse tend to report a worse quality of life and overall poorer health status than women who have not experienced abuse.[6–9,20] Physical sequelae can be divided into central nervous system symptoms, gastrointestinal disorders, cardiac problems, and gynecologic problems. These conditions include, but are not limited to, headaches, seizures, irritable bowel syndrome, sexually transmitted diseases, and vaginal pain.[8,9] As discussed elsewhere in this book (Chapter 14), depression is the most prevalent psychological sequela,[8] followed by posttraumatic stress disorder (PTSD).[21] The more severe the abuse, the more likely a woman is to develop PTSD.[21,22] Other psychological problems associated with IPV include anxiety, insomnia, and substance abuse.[8,21] Gynecologic outcomes, including reproductive problems, are discussed elsewhere (Chapter 7).

Several specific health consequences of IPV are discussed here, including chronic pain syndromes, exacerbation of preexisting disorders, outcomes of insufficient use of the healthcare system, and use of alcohol and drugs. Other outcomes (psychological, reproductive, obstetric) are discussed elsewhere in this book (Chapters 7 and 14).

Chronic Pain Syndromes

Chronic pain syndromes include conditions such as nonspecific headaches, back pain, and fibromyalgia, to name a few, and they are relatively common in survivors.[23] Fibromyalgia and PTSD have been described as occurring together in one study of female survivors of IPV.[24] Sexual and physical abuse have been described in women with fibromyalgia.[25] Physical and sexual abuse rates were approximately the same for those who had fibromyalgia and for those without the condition. However, women with fibromyalgia reported being raped 3.1 times more than women without fibromyalgia.[25]

Exacerbation of Preexisting Conditions

It is not unusual for stress, which IPV certainly represents, to cause certain disorders to flare. For instance, conditions like fibromyalgia, as just noted, may become more difficult to control in an individual subjected to chronic stress.[25] An individual with a chronic disease requiring long-term treatment, such as diabetes or hypertension, may be unable to get the medications she needs because of control of her actions by the abuser, including not getting money to pay for the drugs or not even being allowed to go to the drugstore to get them. Breast cancer exacerbations have been reported in IPV victims as a result of stress,[26] and access to clinical follow-up may be prevented as just noted.

Outcomes Related to Insufficient Use of the Healthcare System

As already noted, a victim may not be permitted to see a doctor or get prescriptions filled or exercise or eat properly because of her abuser's control. Not only will existing diseases not get proper care, but early diagnosis of some conditions may be missed, leading to more severe disease when finally recognized. Studies report that abused women are less likely to get screening or follow-up mammograms[27] or other screening tests. Thus, if they do develop the disease, its detection is likely to occur at a much more advanced and less treatable stage.

Use of Alcohol and Drugs

A number of reports indicate that victims of IPV tend to drink more alcohol, smoke more cigarettes, and use more drugs[28,29] than their nonabused counterparts. An association of drug abuse and sexual abuse by males over time has been reported.[30] However, use of substances of abuse by victims do not represent any failure on the part of the victim, nor can they be proposed as reasons why she gets abused (i.e., the abuse is *not* her fault because she drinks, etc.). Most commonly the use of such agents represents another effort by the victim to ease the burden of her situation, by finding some relief or escape from her daily suffering by attempting to reduce stress through their use. One must refrain from blaming an abused woman who uses alcohol or other addictive agents excessively for being responsible for her abuse (see Chapter 15).

SOCIAL IMPACT OF INTIMATE PARTNER VIOLENCE

Women who have been abused are often at a significant financial disadvantage when they finally get out of the abusive situation. They may not have worked for a long time, they often have no savings or other funds of their own, and they frequently lack certain basics that others take for granted, such as a wardrobe suitable for job interviews. Many advocacy groups and shelters are able to assist women in getting access to job training, legal assistance, and even clothing through a variety of nonprofit agencies. Such resources are available in most communities, but the survivors often need help finding them.

The effect of witnessing domestic violence in the home is a recognized adverse event for children who see such interactions.[31] Some states now have laws increasing the level of the crime of IPV if children witness or even hear a domestic dispute.[32] Some studies have indicated that children who grow up in abusive homes, even if they are not the direct recipients of abuse, are at greater risk for becoming victims or perpetrators when they grow up.[1,33-35] Another potential impact of IPV on society is when the violence spills into the workplace. There are far too many reports in newspapers and in other media of cases in which abusers have gone to the workplace of the victim and not only killed her but other innocent bystanders as well.

REFERENCES

1. NCADV fact sheet. National Coalition Against Domestic Violence Web site. http://www.ncadv.org/files/DomesticViolenceFactSheet(National).pdf. Accessed April 5, 2010.
2. Kyriacou DN, Anglin D, Taliaferro, et al. Risk factors for injury to women from domestic violence against women. *N Engl J Med.* 1999;341:1892–1898.
3. McCauley J, Kern DE, Kolodner K, et al. The "battering syndrome": prevalence and clinical characteristics of domestic violence in primary care internal medicine practices. *Ann Intern Med.* 1995;123:737–746.
4. Alpert EJ. Violence in intimate relationships and the practicing internist: new "disease" or new agenda? *Ann Int Med.* 1995;123:774–781.
5. Eisenstat SA, Bancroft L. Domestic violence. *N Engl J Med.* 1999;341:886–892.
6. Campbell J, Jones AS, Dienemann J, et al. Intimate partner violence and physical health consequences. *Arch Intern Med.* 2002;162:1157–1163.
7. Campbell JC. Health consequences of intimate partner violence. *Lancet.* 2002;359:1331–1336.

8. Coker AL, Davis KE, Arias I, et al. Physical and mental health effects of intimate partner violence for men and women. *Am J Prev Med.* 2002;23:260–268.

9. Coker AL, Smith PH, Bethea L, King MR, McKeown RE. Physical health consequences of physical and psychological intimate partner violence. *Arch Fam Med.* 2000;9:451–457.

10. Chartier MJ, Walker JR, Naimark B. Childhood abuse, adult health, and health care utilization: results from a representative community sample. *Am J Epidemiol.* 2007;165:1031–1038.

11. Baly A. Leaving abusive relationships: constructions of self and situation by abused women [published online ahead of print January 25, 2010]. *J Interpers Violence.* doi: 10.1177/0886260509354885.

12. Filson J, Ulloa E, Runfola C, Hokoda A. Does powerlessness explain the relationship between IPV and depression? *J Interpers Violence.* 2010;25(3):400–415.

13. Wright CV, Collinsworth L, Fitzgerald LF. Why did this happen to me? Cognitive schema disruption and posttraumatic stress disorder in victims of sexual trauma [published online ahead of print December 16, 2009]. doi:10.1177/0886260509354500.

14. Rodriguez MA, Bauer HM, McLoughlin E, Grumback K. Screening and intervention for intimate partner abuse: practices and attitudes of primary care physicians. *JAMA.* 1999;282:468–474.

15. Klap R, Tang L, Wells K, Starks SL, Rodriguez M. Screening for domestic violence among adult women in the US. *J Gen Intern Med.* 2007;22:579–584.

16. Punukollu M. Domestic violence: Screening made practical. *J Fam Pract.* 2003;52:537–543.

17. Neufeld B. SAFE questions: overcoming barriers to the detection of domestic violence. *Am Fam Physician.* 1996;53:2575–2580.

18. Alpert EJ, Albright CL. Domestic violence: screening and documentation. *Hippocrates.* 2000;3:39–43.

19. Fogarty CT, Burge S, McCord EC. Communicating with patients about intimate partner violence: screening and interviewing approaches. *Fam Med.* 2002;34:369–375.

20. Coker AL. Preventing intimate partner violence: how will we rise to this challenge? *Am J Prev Med.* 2006;30:528–529.

21. Woods SJ, Hall RJ, Campbell JC, Angott DM. Physical health and posttraumatic stress disorder symptoms in women experiencing intimate partner violence. *J Midwifery Women's Health.* 2008;53:538–546.

22. Humphreys J, Cooper BA, Miaskowski C. Differences in depression, posttraumatic stress disorder, and lifetime trauma exposure in formerly abused women with mild versus moderate to severe chronic pain [published online ahead of print February 2, 2010]. *J Interpers Violence.* doi:10.1177/0886260509354882.

23. Wuest J, Merritt-Gray M, Ford-Gilboe M, Lent B, Varcoe C, Campbell JC. Chronic pain in women survivors of intimate partner violence. *J Pain.* 2008;9:1049–1057.

24. Raphael KG, Janal MN, Nayak S. Comorbidity of fibromyalgia and posttraumatic stress disorder symptoms in a community sample of women. *Pain Med.* 2004;5:33–41.

25. Ciccone DS, Elliott DK, Chandler HK, Nayak S, Raphael KG. Sexual and physical abuse in women with fibromyalgia syndrome: a test of the trauma hypothesis. *Clin J Pain.* 2005;21:378–386.

26. Deimling GT, Bowman KF, Sterms S, Wagner LJ, Kahana B. Cancer-related health worries and psychological distress among older adult, long-term cancer survivors. *Psychooncology.* 2006;15(4):306–320.

27. Moy B, Park ER, Feibelmann S, Chiang S, Weissman JS. Barriers to repeat mammography: cultural perspectives of African American, Asian, and Hispanic women. *Psychooncology.* 2006;15:623–634.

28. Zinzo HM, Resnick HS, Amstadter AB, McCauley JL, Ruggiero KJ, Kilpatrick, DG. Drug- or alcohol-facilitated, incapacitated, and forcible rape in relationship to mental health among a national sample of women [published online ahead of print January 25, 2010]. *J Interpers Violence.* doi:10.1177/0886260509354887.

29. Brecklin LR, Ullman SE. The roles of victim and offender substance use in sexual assault outcomes. *J Interpers Violence.* 2010;25(8):1503–1522.

30. Swartout KM, White JW. The relationship between drug use and sexual aggression in men across time. *J Interpers Violence.* 2010;25(9):1716–1735.

31. Edleson JL. Problems associated with children's witnessing of domestic violence. April 1999. Available at http://www.unified-solutions.org/uploads/problemswithchildwitnessdv.pdf. Accessed April 15, 2010.

32. Alaska Stat. § 47.17.035 (1998), Ind. Code § 5-2-9-2.1 (1998), and S.D. Codified Laws § 26-7A-107 (1996) as cited by Mathews, M. Available at http://www.policyforresults.org/ en/Topics/2008/Building-Strong-and-Stable-Families/State-Child-Welfare-Policy-Guide/1/Families/Preserving-and-Reunifying-Families/Removal-of-the-perpetrator.aspx. Accessed April 14, 2010.

33. Luthra R, Abramovitz R, Greenberg R, et al. Relationship between type of trauma exposure and post-traumatic stress disorder among urban children and adolescents. *J Interpers Violence.* 2009;24(11):1919–1927.

34. Afifi TO, Ennis MW, Cox BJ, Asmundson GJ, Stein MB, Sareen J. Population attributable fractions of psychiatric disorders and suicide ideation and attempts associated with adverse childhood experiences. *Am J Public Health.* 2008;98(5): 946–952.

35. Teicher MH, Samson JA, Polcari A, McGreenery CE. Sticks, stones, and hurtful words: relative effects of various forms of childhood maltreatment. *Am J Psychiatry.* 2006;163(6):993–1000.

Intimate Partner Violence and Women's Reproductive Health

Sarina Schrager, MD, MS

INTRODUCTION

Intimate partner violence (IPV) has many implications for women's reproductive health. IPV has been related to increased risks of sexually transmitted infections (STIs) and human immunodeficiency virus (HIV), lack of fertility control for women, adverse pregnancy outcomes, and increased rates of cervical cancer. This chapter reviews the evidence linking IPV in heterosexual relationships and the reproductive health of women. There are significant reproductive health differences between women in Western countries and women in developing countries, including HIV rates and use of contraception. The data reviewed focus on women in developed countries.

The theoretical basis for a relationship between STIs or HIV and IPV stems from the inequality of the relationship between the female and male partners. The dynamics of the power differential enables the male partner to dominate the female partner and make decisions for her. These decisions may relate to her sexuality, her use of contraception, or her fertility. Forced sexual intercourse, a specific type of sexual IPV, is associated with multiple gynecologic problems, including STIs, chronic pelvic pain, and dyspareunia.[1]

Decisions regarding how and when to have sexual intercourse or whether to use condoms often are made by the male partner (perpetrator of IPV in this model).

SEXUALLY TRANSMITTED INFECTION AND HUMAN IMMUNODEFICIENCY VIRUS

IPV is associated with risky sexual behaviors, including inconsistent condom use, that likely contribute to the increased risk of STIs in general.[2] Seventeen of the 24 studies included in a 2007 systematic review found that women with a history of IPV had higher rates of STIs.[2] Seven contributors to increased risk of HIV in female victims of IPV were described by El-Bassel et al.[3]

1. Engaging in unprotected sex
2. Higher rates of other STIs
3. Sex with multiple partners
4. Engaging in unprotected anal sex
5. Positive HIV status of the partner
6. Trading sex for drugs
7. Having a risky sexual partner

In a cohort of women on methadone in New York, those with a history of IPV were less likely to use condoms regularly.[3]

A large epidemiologic study of women in the United States ($n = 13,928$) found that a woman's experience of IPV in the past year was significantly associated with her risk of being HIV positive (relative risk [RR]: 3.44; 95% confidence interval [CI]: 1.28–9.22).[4] In further analysis of their data, the researchers estimated that 11.8% of the HIV cases were directly related to the occurrence of IPV.[4] A cohort of married women from India ($n = 28,139$) were asked about IPV risk and tested for HIV. Experiencing both physical and sexual IPV was associated with a significant increase in the risk of HIV (odds ratio [OR]: 3.92; 95% CI: 1.41–10.94; $p = 0.01$) in that population.[5]

CONTRACEPTION AND FERTILITY CONTROL

When the male partner makes the decisions about sexuality and contraception, women may have less ability to control their own fertility. In a cross-sectional survey given to young women (ages 16–29 years) attending family planning clinics in California ($n = 1278$), 19% of the respondents admitted to pregnancy coercion (being forced to become pregnant) and 15% admitted to contraceptive sabotage (i.e., holes in condoms or diaphragms, or promising to "pull out" but not doing it).[6] This same study found that both pregnancy coercion and contraceptive sabotage were associated with unintended pregnancies (adjusted odds ratio [AOR] 1.83; 95% CI: 1.36–2.46 and AOR: 1.58; 95% CI: 1.14–2.20, respectively).[6] A written survey of more than 1400 women in Philadelphia found that IPV was consistently associated with a woman's partner's unwillingness to use contraception, his making the use of contraception difficult, and his desire for pregnancy.[7] In this study, IPV was associated with higher numbers of pregnancies, with each additional pregnancy associated with a 10% increased risk of IPV.[7] A case-control study of 225 women found that women who experienced physical or emotional IPV were less likely to use the contraception that they wanted (OR: 1.9, 95% CI: 1.0–3.7).[8]

Inconsistent contraceptive use and unintended pregnancies may lead to increased abortion rates as well. More than 300 women requesting an abortion at a clinic in England were questioned about their history of IPV. In this sample, 19.5% had experienced physical abuse in the past year, and 3.7% had endured forced sexual intercourse.[9] An older study of more than 400 women in North Carolina at an abortion clinic found that more than 39% of them had experienced abuse.[10] Women with abuse histories were less likely to inform their partner (often the abuser) about the pregnancy than women who had not been abused.[10] A similar study of 62 women attending an abortion clinic in New Zealand found a 43% lifetime prevalence of physical abuse and a 32% lifetime prevalence of sexual abuse.[11] A qualitative study that included interviews with eight pregnant women requesting abortions who were victims of abuse explored women's fears that if they had the babies the violence would continue and possibly worsen.[12]

PREGNANCY COMPLICATIONS

Abused women who choose to keep their pregnancies may be at higher risk of a myriad of antenatal, intrapartum, and postpartum conditions (Chapter 11). IPV has been linked to increased rates of STIs in pregnancy and an increased risk of preterm labor and preterm delivery.[13] A 2004 systematic review of 30 articles on this subject also found that IPV was related to multiple adverse pregnancy outcomes, including low birthweight and small for gestational age infants, more frequent kidney infections, and increased maternal mortality.[14] The risk of maternal mortality in abused mothers was three times that of nonabused mothers.[14] IPV-related homicide may account for some of the difference in mortality.[15] A retrospective study of police-reported IPV incidents in pregnant women in Seattle found that women who were victims of IPV during pregnancy had higher antenatal hospitalization rates when compared with a cohort of nonabused pregnant women (AOR: 2.39; 95%

CI: 1.77–3.24).[16] In addition, abused pregnant women are less likely to obtain prenatal care and are more likely to smoke and use drugs during their pregnancies, both of which can lead to adverse pregnancy outcomes.[15]

Experiences of IPV also have been associated with higher rates of cervical cancer, likely due to unprotected intercourse and exposure to IPV. One study of more than 4200 women in Kentucky found that after adjusting for other factors, ever experiencing IPV was associated with a significantly increased risk of having invasive cervical cancer (AOR: 2.6; 95% CI: 1.7–3.9).[17] IPV also may contribute to treatment adherence after a cancer diagnosis.[18]

In all, IPV has many effects on women's reproductive health. These may be direct (e.g., forced sexual intercourse) or indirect (from controlling behavior). Clinicians should ask women about their history of IPV in an effort to determine effective contraception and STI risk. Clinicians may counsel women who are in abusive relationships to use "invisible" methods of contraception like depomedroxyprogesterone acetate injections or an intrauterine device. In addition, clinicians should consider female victims of IPV at high risk for STIs and HIV and should screen accordingly.

REFERENCES

1. Campbell JC. Health consequences of intimate partner violence. *Lancet.* 2002;359:1331–1336.
2. Coker AL. Does physical intimate partner violence affect sexual health? A systematic review. *Trauma Violence Abuse.* 2007;8(2):149–177.
3. El-Bassel N, Gilbert L, Wu E, Go H, Hill J. HIV and intimate partner violence among methadone-maintained women in New York City. *Soc Sci Med.* 2005;61:171–183.
4. Sareen J, Pagura J, Grant B. Is intimate partner violence associated with HIV infection among women in the United States? *Gen Hosp Psychiatry.* 2009;31(3): 274–278.
5. Silverman JG, Decker MR, Saggurti N, Balaiah D, Raj A. Intimate partner violence and HIV infection among married Indian women. *JAMA.* 2008;300(6):703–710.
6. Miller E, Decker MR, McCauley HL, et al. Pregnancy coercion, intimate partner violence, and unintended pregnancy. *Contraception.* 2010;81(4):316–322.
7. Gee RE, Mitra N, Wan F, Chavkin DE, Long JA. Power over parity: intimate partner violence and issues of fertility control. *Am J Obstet Gynecol.* 2009;201:148.e1–7.
8. Williams CM, Larsen U, McCloskey LA. Intimate partner violence and women's contraceptive use. *Violence Against Women.* 2008;14(12):1382–1396.
9. Keeling J, Birch L. The prevalence rates of domestic abuse in women attending a family planning clinic. *J Fam Plann Reprod Health Care.* 2004;30(2):113–114.
10. Glander SS, Moore ML, Michielutte R, Parsons LH. The prevalence of domestic violence among women seeking abortion. *Obstet Gynecol.* 1998;91(6):1002–1006.
11. Whitehead A, Fanslow J. Prevalence of family violence amongst women attending an abortion clinic in New Zealand. *Aust NZ J Obstet Gynaecol.* 2005;45(4):321–324.

12. Williams GB, Brackley MH. Intimate partner violence, pregnancy and the decision for abortion. *Issues Ment Health Nurs.* 2009;30(4):272–278.

13. Sharps PW, Laughon K, Giangrande SK. Intimate partner violence and the childbearing year: maternal and infant consequences. *Trauma Violence Abuse.* 2007;8(2):105–116.

14. Boy A, Salihu HM. Intimate partner violence and birth outcomes: a systematic review. *Int J Fertil Womens Med.* 2004;49(4):159–164.

15. Chambliss LR. Intimate partner violence and its implication for pregnancy. *Clin Obstet Gynecol.* 2008;51(2):385–397.

16. Lipsky S, Holt VL, Easterling TR, Critchlow CW. Police-reported intimate partner violence during pregnancy and the risk of antenatal hospitalization. *Matern Child Health J.* 2004;8(2):55–63.

17. Coker AL, Hopenhayn C, DeSimone CP, Bush HM, Crofford L. Violence against women raises risk of cervical cancer. *J Womens Health (Larchmt).* 2009;18(8):1179–1185.

18. Martino MM, Balar A, Cragun JM, Hoffman MS. Delay in treatment of invasive cervical cancer due to intimate partner violence. *Gynecol Oncol.* 2005;99:507–509.

Chapter 8

Intimate Partner Violence in Same-Sex Relationships

Kathy Oriel, MD, MS

INTRODUCTION

Abusive control of an intimate partner is not a strategy employed solely by heterosexual dyads. Whether tactics are physical, sexual, or psychological, perpetrators use similar approaches to denigrate and belittle, whether straight or gay. Uncovering intimate partner violence (IPV) within same-sex relationships may be even more difficult than the challenging task of identifying victims in heterosexual relationships. Once the evidence of an abusive dynamic is irrefutable, obtaining support and resources for victims leads to another array of unique struggles.

Same-sex orientation may refer to sexual attraction, sexual contact, or an intimate emotional relationship between partners of the same gender. For most lesbian woman and gay men, their sexual attraction, sexual contact, and intimate emotional relationships are aligned, yet for others this is not the case. For example, a woman may have intimate emotional connection and attraction to another woman and never act sexually on it, or a man may identify as heterosexual but have occasional sexual contact with men. Neither of these individuals may identify themselves as lesbian or gay. Further, many gay men and lesbian women have had intimate emotional and sexual relationships with members of the opposite gender in the past. Same-sex IPV (SSIPV) refers to verbal threats or intimidation, physical assault, or forced sexual contact within an intimate emotional and sexual relationship.

PREVALENCE

The United States Department of Justice (DOJ) and Centers for Disease Control and Prevention (CDC) co-sponsored the National Violence Against Women Survey (NVAW),[1] and the research report was published in 2000. The NVAW consisted of a nationally representative sample of 8000 US women and 8000 US men addressing experiences as victims of violence. This survey addressed many facets of IPV and specifically queried whether respondents had ever lived with a same-sex partner as part of a couple. The survey obtained the gender of perpetrators, which allowed researchers to compare populations of same-sex and heterosexual couples. In this sample, only 1% of women ($n = 79$) and 0.8% of men ($n = 65$) reported living with a same-sex intimate partner at least once during their lifetime. These women, who at some time lived "as a couple" with another woman, should arguably represent a subset of the lesbian population in this sample. Among these lesbian women, 11.4% reported being victimized by a female partner, but 30% of the same women reported being victimized by a male partner in the past. Women who reported cohabitating only with men (arguably a subset of the heterosexual population) were victimized at a rate of 20.3% or almost twice that of the same-sex cohabitors.

Men in this study who partnered or cohabited at some time in their lives with another man were similarly more likely to be victimized by a male partner than by a female partner. Among these same-sex cohabitors, 15.4% reported being raped, physically assaulted, and/or stalked by a male partner, whereas 10.8% of these men experienced such violence at the hands of a female perpetrator. Men who coupled and cohabitated heterosexually reported victimization at the hands of their female partners at a rate of 7.7%, half the rate that same-sex male partners experienced. These NVAW findings would suggest that men are more likely to perpetrate violence whether heterosexually or homosexually partnered.

Greenwood et al[2] used a somewhat complicated sampling technique to obtain a representative gay male sample and evaluate for SSIPV. These researchers predicted high-density gay male neighborhoods using data from men-who-have-sex-with-men (MSM) AIDS cases, commercial gay mailing lists, and 1990 census data on male-male-partnered households in four large cities. They constructed a random-digit dialing sample for designated telephone prefixes, then oversampled these "higher gay density" neighborhoods. Only one man from each household was interviewed, and of the 3700 eligible men, 2881 completed phone interviews. Respondents were asked to report "unwanted physical or emotional violence" from a boyfriend over the past 5 years, using a modified Conflict Tactics Scale (CTS). This study revealed that 34% of these gay men experienced emotional abuse from a partner over the past 5 years. Among this group, 22% experienced physical abuse, and 5% were sexually assaulted by an intimate partner. Younger age independently predicted higher rates of abuse, and HIV-seropositive men were 1.5 times as likely to experience multiple batterings when compared with HIV-negative men.[2]

Representative sampling within the lesbian, gay, bisexual, transgender, and queer (LGBTQ) population remains a substantial barrier to all public health efforts within this community but is even more problematic in the area of partner abuse. Attempts to define and understand IPV in same-sex relationships have typically used convenience samples of self-identified lesbians or gay men. Some used "snowball" survey techniques where initial participants are asked to refer other friends and acquaintances to participate.[3] Most published studies have surveyed gays and lesbians through known gay venues, such as bars, gay pride events, social organizations, or mailing lists. Burke and Follingstad[3] notes that these techniques oversample urban, younger, drinking, and extroverted gays and lesbians. These respondents also tend to lack a consistent sexual partner. Reviews by Burke and Follingstad[3]and Murray and Mobley[4] summarize this literature and delineate the limitations of studies aspiring to describe the scope of the problem. These sampling limitations, linked with inconsistent tools to define abuse, result in broad and conflicting estimates of SSIPV prevalence, although most suspect rates are similar to those in heterosexual couples.

Convenience samples may result in reporting bias in that victims may be more likely to return surveys or may systematically not return them due to fear of retribution. Most studies do not elucidate whether violence was inflicted in self-defense. Convenience samples also may include both members of a couple, resulting in an unintentional doubling of prevalence data. These samples are commonly recruited from mailing lists or music festivals and thus should not be generalized to the lesbian and gay population at large, and prevalence rates from these convenience samples should not be compared with heterosexual rates of IPV from population-based samples.[2-4]

Previous studies on SSIPV did not specifically query gender of the perpetrator, so if the woman identified as lesbian and reported a history of abuse as an adult, that perpetrator could have been assumed to be female, when in fact it was a prior male partner who was abusive.[4] Finally, as in other IPV research, large differences exist among investigators when defining IPV. Although some studies use well-validated, specific behavioral instruments like the Conflict Tactics Scale (CTS),[5] others use terminology such as *abused*, which is known to decrease response rates because many individuals who are pushed, shoved, hit, or verbally assaulted often do not define those behaviors as abuse.[5]

UNIQUE ISSUES IN SAME-SEX INTIMATE PARTNER VIOLENCE

The National Coalition of Anti-Violence Programs (NCAVP) provides national advocacy for local lesbian, gay, bisexual, and transgendered communities. The NCAVP serves as a network of "over 35 anti-violence organizations that monitor, respond to, and work to end hate and domestic violence."[6] Each year, local organizations collect data that "addresses the pervasive problem of violence committed against and within the LGBTQ and HIV-positive communities."[6] These annual reports include personal anecdotes and identify some of the challenges unique to those in same-sex violent relationships.

Homophobia and Threats of "Outing"

Abusers in same-sex relationships sometimes threaten partners who contemplate leaving the pairing with "outing" them, or telling others that they are lesbian or gay. Gays and lesbians, whether victimized or not, may hide their sexual orientation from others. Not being open about one's primary relationship or sexual orientation is referred to as being "in the closet." Many lesbians, gays, and bisexuals fear job discrimination, losing custody of children, or alienation from family and friends. Others maintain a sense of shame or embarrassment about their sexual orientation. For someone who is both closeted and abused, sharing sexual orientation and victim status is simply more than she or he can bear. Individuals who are openly gay may fear telling others about their abusive relationship because they fear this may reinforce cultural stereotypes that gays and lesbians are mentally ill or that all same-sex relationships are fundamentally dysfunctional.[3]

Gays and lesbians receive societal messages that they are morally repugnant, should be religiously scorned, or their relationships are less desirable and valuable than those of their heterosexual peers. When gays and lesbians believe these messages about themselves and fear others will not like or respect them if they tell the truth about their orientation, this is internalized homophobia. Internalized homophobia may contribute to increased health risk behaviors and may result in victims believing that they deserve poor treatment.[3]

Social Support

Some lesbians and gays may have weaker social support systems than their heterosexual peers. Despite increasing acceptance in recent years, many lesbian women and gay men are still estranged from their families. Others move away from the communities where they were raised to be in cities with larger numbers of gay people. When a social safety net is already dangerously thin, staying with an abusive partner may appear superior to being completely alone.

Misperception That Abuse Is Mutual or Equal

Same-sex partners lack the societal power differential often present in heterosexual couples. Similarly, the common size and strength disparities typically found in straight couples leads some to view physical violence, verbal intimidation, or forced sexual behavior between two men or two women as more acceptable or mutual. The NCAVP defines IPV as "a pattern of behavior where one intimate partner coerces, dominates, and isolates the other intimate partner in order to maintain power and control over the partner and over the relationship."[6] Advocates, mental health professionals, and survivors themselves describe familiar dynamics in same-sex battery: an unrelenting drive for power and control, repeated cycles of abuse and reconciliation, escalation of violence over time, and increased risk for victims when they attempt to leave the relationship. These characteristics are indistinguishable from IPV in heterosexual couples (Chapter 3).

Ability of Perpetrator to Claim He or She Is the Victim

Advocates and community workers involved in programs for victims of SSIPV have long described incidents where both partners of a couple present to shelters or advocacy groups claiming victimization. The NCAVP[6] documents incidents where an abuse survivor was arrested because the abuser made claims of victimization.

Although some abuse survivors and community advocates express fear that the police may disproportionately arrest both partners in a same-sex domestic incident, Pattavina et al[7] obtained data from the National Incident-Based Reporting System, containing more than 176,000 intimate partner assaults and intimidation incidents in 19 reporting states during 2000. The researchers were interested in determining whether similar cases involving same-sex and heterosexual couples resulted in similar police response. Same-sex couples were identified in 1077 cases, or fewer than 1%, and incidents involving same-sex couples were equally likely to result in an arrest. As anticipated, the more serious the offense, the more likely the arrest in both groups. The other major predictor of arrest likelihood was state-specific legislation directing police on how to handle domestic incidents. The effect of "mandatory arrest" laws and increased likelihood of arrest was similar in heterosexual and same-sex couples, suggesting that in these reporting states police are consistent in applying the arrest law.

Misperception That the Physically Larger, More Masculine Partner (More "Butch") Is Likely to be the Perpetrator

Domestic violence education has historically focused on heterosexual couples where the man is more likely to be abusive and is commonly physically larger and stronger. This had led some to assume the larger or more masculine partner (whether the same-sex couple is male or female) is the perpetrator. Dynamics of power in same-sex situations are more complicated, and the assumption that perpetrator and victim can be determined based on physical appearance or gender is wrong.

Repercussions in the Gay Community

Although advocacy groups and attention to SSIPV have grown since the early 1990s, many acknowledge that the gay community has been slow to highlight SSIPV as a health priority for the LGBTQ community. Some fear that open acknowledgment of IPV within gay and lesbian relationships could be used as evidence that gay and lesbian relationships are inherently unhealthy and do not deserve legal protections, such as marriage. This neglect may contribute to further isolation of victims within the only community where their relationship is acknowledged and celebrated. Victims seeking LGBTQ-specific resources agonize that in a smaller tight-knit community the abuser will immediately know his or her whereabouts or be notified of his or her attempts to gain freedom.

RESOURCES FOR VICTIMS

Accessing domestic violence resources for men has been historically challenging. Shelters were commonly not welcoming of lesbian women, so victims fleeing abusive home situations felt they had to lie about the gender of their abuser to gain safe haven. Similarly, shelters and advocacy organizations were slow to conceptualize men as victims.

The National Coalition of Anti-Violence Programs (ncavp.org) lists local services for LGBTQ victims of violence, whether victimized by a partner or a stranger. These 15 programs specifically address the needs of same-sex victims, as well as providing resources for perpetrators, are all located in urban areas. Telephone hotlines serve those in any geographic location.

These local advocacy groups track shelters and other advocacy groups that are open and accepting to gay men and lesbian women.

Aardvarc is a nonprofit educational and advocacy agency that stands for An Abuse, Rape, Domestic Violence Aid and Resource Collection. The Aardvarc Web site (http://www.aardvarc.org/dv/gay.shtml) outlines common myths and provides a myriad of resources, including books and popular press resources about same-sex IPV.

LEGAL PROTECTION FOR VICTIMS OF SAME-SEX INTIMATE PARTNER VIOLENCE

Although a handful of states narrowly define IPV as only occurring between a man and a woman who have been married or cohabiting, many states have crafted language in IPV statutes that ensure gender neutrality. This language affords protection for victims of IPV who have lived with or had an intimate dating relationship with someone, regardless of gender. Other states do not specifically define parties involved in IPV either way. Illinois, Ohio, Kentucky, and Hawaii have laws that specifically allow victims in same-sex relationships to obtain a restraining order. Montana, Arizona, New York, Delaware, Louisiana, South Carolina, and Virginia have laws that specifically deny victims from receiving an order of protection. Florida, Mississippi, and Maryland have laws that are ambiguous but could exclude victims of SSIPV.[8] All other states have laws that are gender neutral and do not specifically include or exclude gay and lesbian couples in their statutes.

APPLICATION IN THE CLINICAL SETTING

Screening

No studies have specifically investigated whether there are any differences in screening for IPV in same-sex couples in comparison to heterosexual couples. McClennen et al[9] developed a "Lesbian Partner Abuse Scale," but even the revised version at 29 items was not designed for clinical screening. A few simple common-sense approaches can help LGBTQ individuals feel welcome and safe in clinical settings. First, providers should be trained never to assume patients are heterosexual. People of all ages, races, ethnicities, and appearance may have same-sex behaviors or identities. Although some persons do have stereotypical appearance or mannerisms, no one, including the lesbian or gay clinician, should rely on "gaydar," the slang term gays and lesbians use when they sense someone else is gay. Clinicians should invariably use gender-inclusive language, such as "Do you have a life partner?" or

"Do you date men, women, both, or neither?" This inclusive language signals to the patient that it is safe to disclose a same-sex relationship. When screening for IPV, similar gender-neutral language in using any of the office-based screening questions is imperative:

- Within the past year, have you been hit, slapped, kicked, or physically hurt by someone?
- Does your partner, or someone you are dating, ever threaten you or pressure you to participate in sexual activity that makes you uncomfortable?

Lesbian women in abusive relationships do seek help from formal sources about 60% of the time and from informal sources approximately 80% of the time, rates similar to heterosexual women in abusive relationships.[3] Creation of a nonjudgmental office environment will ideally facilitate disclosure to clinicians and mental health professionals. Few studies have explored help-seeking behaviors in same-sex couples, and none are recent. Lie and Gentlewarrier[10] reported that lesbian survivors sought help most frequently from private therapy and counseling, support groups specifically for battered lesbians, self-help groups, and battered women's shelters.

TREATMENT AND RESOURCES FOR BATTERERS

Bradford and colleagues[11] reported that lesbian perpetrators sought help from the same resources as heterosexual women victims except for battered women's shelters. Medical facilities, clergy, police, and women's organizations were found to be less helpful. Margolies and Leeder[12] reported on a group of 30 lesbian perpetrators in the 1990s. They analyzed the psychological profiles of these women and determined that the abusers tended to be enmeshed and overly dependent on their partners, suggesting that these women battered in a misguided attempt to avoid abandonment. These authors treated abusers with a combination of group therapy for urban participants and individual couple and community approaches for rural women. In this descriptive paper, they used anger management skills and addressed common coping techniques. In 2003, Coleman[13] described specific psychotherapeutic techniques useful in treating lesbian batterers. These techniques are based in personality development theory and use attachment theory, affect regulation, and work on internalized homophobia and vindictiveness. Treatment of lesbian batterers via common court-ordered treatment modalities would likely place the female perpetrator in a group of male batterers that is not designed for the unique underlying issues in lesbian battering. Washington State, Massachusetts,[14] and California have developed lesbian and gay batterer intervention programs, and all incorporate work on homophobia in addition to the usual dynamics addressed in such programs. Data on the outcomes from these programs, if available at all, are not readily accessible.

IPV is common in lesbian and gay relationships and carries with it unique barriers beyond the already complex social, psychological, medical, and spiritual issues manifest with all IPV. Despite a field that has existed in the literature for more than 30 years, a paltry sum of data informs our practice regarding SSIPV. Evaluating the role that homophobia, racism, classism, and other oppressions impart on individuals, and how these oppressions influence coping and recovery, has not been adequately addressed but seems imperative. We need to understand how identities as gay man or lesbian woman, adult survivor, child abuse survivor, substance user, racial or ethnic minority, transgendered person, or socioeconomic status affects each individual. If anything, the last 30 years have taught us that the gay and lesbian communities are resilient and resourceful. Like many other issues facing this group, activists have created the community-specific resources to best meet the needs of their people. These agents of social change and advocacy must now share outcomes and lessons with others to produce true progress. Once the evidence exists and is reported, we must use it to advise legislative agendas, public health policy, and medical practice in a way that decreases the burden of violence for all people.

REFERENCES

1. Tjaden P, Thoennes N. Extent, nature, and consequence of intimate partner violence: findings from the National Violence Against Women Survey. Washington, DC: U.S. Department of Justice, National Institute of Justice; July 2000. NCJ181867.
2. Greenwood GL, Relf MV, Huang B, et al. Battering victimization among a probability-based sample of men who have sex with men. *Am J Public Health.* 2002:92:1964–1969.
3. Burke LK, Follingstad DR. Violence in lesbian and gay relationships: theory, prevalence, and correlational factors. *Clin Psychol Rev.* 1999;19:487–512.
4. Murray CE, Mobley AK. Empirical research about same-sex intimate partner violence: a methodological review. *J Homosexuality.* 2009;56:361–386.
5. Straus MA. Measuring intrafamily conflict and violence: The conflict tactics (CT) scales. *J Marriage Fam.* 1979;41:75–88.
6. Fountain K, Mitchell-Brody M, Jones S, Nichols K. *Lesbian, Gay, Bisexual, Transgender and Queer Domestic Violence in the United States in 2008.* A report from the National Coalition of Anti-Violence Programs. NCAVP Web site. http://www.avp.org/documents/2008NCAVPLGBTQDVReportFINAL.pdf. Accessed September 9, 2010.
7. Pattavina A, Hirschel D, Buzawa E, et al. A comparison of the police response to heterosexual versus same-sex intimate partner violence. *Violence Against Women.* 2007;13:374–394.

8. Barnes PG. It's just a quarrel. *Am Bar Assoc J.* 1998;84:24–25.

9. McClennen JC, Summer AB, Daley JG. The lesbian partner abuse scale. *Res Soc Work Pract.* 2002;12:277–292.

10. Lie GY, Gentlewarrier S. Intimate violence in lesbian relationships: discussion of survey findings and practice implications. *J Soc Service Res.* 1991;15:41–59.

11. Bradford J, Ryan C, Rothblum ED. National lesbian health care survey: Implications for mental health care. *J Consult Clin Psychol.* 1994;62:228–242.

12. Margolies L, Leeder E. Violence at the door: treatment of lesbian batterers. *Violence Against Women.* 1995;1:139–157.

13. Coleman VE. Treating the lesbian batterer. *J Aggression Maltreat Trauma.* 2003;7: 159–205.

14. Pilot program specifications for intervention with lesbian, gay, bisexual and transgender perpetrators of intimate partner violence. Commonwealth of Massachusetts, Office of Health and Human Services Web site. http://www. mass.gov/Eeohhs2/docs/dph/com_health/violence/bi_guidelines_glbt.pdf. Accessed September 9, 2010.

Chapter 9

Intimate Partner Violence in Women with Disabilities

Deborah Dreyfus, MD

Women with disabilities are at increased risk of interpersonal violence.[1] These women frequently suffer silently because either they do not know where to turn or they are too scared to tell anyone. Many may not even know what is considered abuse. These issues seriously impact the quality of life, and often the very life, of women with physical and intellectual disabilities. Physical disabilities refer to conditions that "substantially limit one or more basic physical activities, such as walking, climbing stairs, reaching, lifting, or carrying."[1] Intellectual disabilities (ID) refer to people who have limitations in intellectual functioning and in adaptive behavior, such as bathing and dressing oneself.[2] The term ID has replaced the older descriptor of "mental retardation."

Types of abuse specific to women with disabilities include withholding needed equipment (e.g., removing a battery from a wheelchair), medications, transportation, and personal assistance services.[3-5] Additionally, women with both physical and intellectual disabilities depend on others to complete many of their activities of daily living. Withholding aid or not providing nutrition is a form of abuse, namely neglect, that is common in women with disabilities.[6-8]

RISK FACTORS

Physical Disabilities

Table 9-1 lists the risk factors for abuse in women with physical disabilities. Of note, limited mobility, social isolation, and personal history of depression are related to increased rates of abuse in women with physical disabilities.

Table 9-1 Risk Factors for the Perpetration of Violence in Women with Physical Disabilities

Individual risk factors
- Younger age
- Decreased mobility
- Social isolation
- Lower socioeconomic status
- High stress level
- Depression
- Short duration relationship
- Previous history of abuse
- Single versus married (single is higher)
- Nonwhite versus white

Risk factors for abusers
- Alcohol/drug use
- Stress

Source: Data from Coker A, Smith PH, Fadden MK. Intimate partner violence and disabilities among women attending family practice clinics. *J Womens Health (Larchmt)*. 2005;14(9):829–838; Nosek M, Hughes R, Taylor H, Taylor P. Disability, psychosocial, and demographic characteristics of abused women with physical disabilities. *Violence Against Women*. 2006;12(9):838–850; Martin S, Ray N, Sotres-Alvarez D, et al. Physical and sexual assault of women with disabilities. *Violence Against Women*. 2006;12(9):823–837; Nosek MEA. Disability, psychosocial, and demographic characteristics of abused women with physical disabilities. *Violence Against Women*. 2006;12(9): 838–850; Martin S, Ray N, Sotres-Alvarez D, et al. Physical and sexual assault of women with disabilities. *Violence Against Women*. 2006;12(9):823–837; McFarlane J, Hughes RB, Nosek MA, Groff JY, Swedlend N, Dolan Mullen P. Abuse assessment screen-disability (AAS-D): Measuring frequency, type, and perpetrator of abuse toward women with physical disabilities. *J Womens Health Gend Based Med*. 2001;10(9):861–866.

Intellectual Disabilities

Women with ID are vulnerable to abuse for many of the same reasons as women with physical disabilities. First, adults with ID often are taught to be compliant, and some may be dependent on others for long-term care. Second, those with ID may not have received education on sexuality and thus may not have learned language that allows them to describe sexual abuse. Third, they often do not even have economic independence and must rely on those around them, possibly the abuser, for care. This may cause fear of reporting the perpetrator: The act of reporting may cause more violence, the loss of housing, or the loss of care on which she relies. Fourth, those being abused may not know how or when to seek justice.[9] In fact, even if abuse is reported, the victim often is thought to be fabricating the complaint.[10] Women with ID may not be able to distinguish between normal behavior and abusive behavior. Finally, those with ID often desire social acceptance and want to be "liked" by those around them. They may allow abusers easier access to commit abuse because of this need to be liked.[10] The act of portraying those with disabilities as vulnerable may actually help contribute to abuse. Many perpetrators choose victims based on this vulnerability, which makes them more likely to become victims.[11]

EPIDEMIOLOGY OF PHYSICAL AND SEXUAL ABUSE

Several studies have examined abuse of women with disabilities without distinguishing between physical and intellectual disabilities. A longitudinal study in Canada evaluated a total of between 6000 and 8000 women with and without disabilities in 1993, 1999, and 2004.[12] The women with disabilities described significantly higher rates of abuse than their non-disabled counterparts. The only differences in risks between the two groups were partner characteristics. Abusive partners of women with disabilities were more likely to be dominant, possessive, and jealous.[12] A 2006 study of more than 23,000 women (6300 with a disability) also found that women with disabilities were significantly more likely to have experienced intimate partner violence (IPV) than the women without disabilities (33.2% vs 21.2%).[13] In this study, women who had experienced IPV had lower self-rated health status and were more likely to have an unmet health need than nondisabled women.[13]

Physical Disabilities

In the general population, as well as in women with disabilities, most abuse is perpetrated by men who have intimate relationships with the victim. A 1997 community-based survey of more than 400 women with a physical disability found that 13% of the women reported physical or sexual abuse by an intimate partner in the past year.[14] However, significant numbers of abusers have relationships with disabled women that are directly related to the disability. For instance, a 1992 review of 162 cases of abuse in women with physical disabilities found that in 44% of the cases abusers were personal care assistants, healthcare providers, residential staff members, transportation providers, foster parents, and other individuals with disabilities.[8] Abuse in women with physical disabilities is more severe than in the general population.[15] In one study, the prevalence of violence (physical, emotional, and sexual) appeared to be the same for those with and without physical disabilities; however, the abuse lasted longer in the group with physical disabilities.[16] Physical and emotional abuse are typically perpetrated by husbands and live-in partners, followed, in decreasing numbers, by mothers, fathers, healthcare workers, and personal care attendants. However, sexual abuse of women with physical disabilities is most commonly perpetrated by strangers.[17]

Intellectual Disabilities

Although women with physical disabilities appear to experience the same rate of abuse as those without disabilities, in some studies the prevalence of abuse in women with ID is higher. In a survey of 511 women with ID from five subspecialty health clinics, 10% were abused in the previous year. The most common perpetrator was an intimate partner, followed by family members and then healthcare providers.[18] Additionally, in three studies of women with ID, lifetime prevalence of sexual abuse alone ranged from 25% to 53%.[18] A 2000 Australian study found that adults with ID are 2.9 times more likely to be physically assaulted and 10.7 times more likely to be sexually assaulted than women in the general population.[9] The authors also reported that in Australia 40% of crimes against people with mild ID and 71% of those with severe ID, again women, went unreported to the police.[9]

Neglect represents one of the most common forms of abuse among women with ID. In a record review of 9400 institutionalized men and women in 23 residential homes in the southern United States, members of the residential staff abused approximately 5% of the residents during the 22-month study; of those who were abused, 43% suffered from neglect and 38% from physical abuse.[17]

EVALUATION

Physical Disabilities

Even if they are able to recognize the abuse, many women do not know where to turn. In addition, many battered women's programs do not have adequate facilities to help women with physical disabilities. A survey of 598 such programs found that less than 1% of the women clients who seek help had physical disabilities.[19] Only 35% of the programs surveyed offered disability awareness training, and only 16% had a staff member with training in disabilities.[19]

Healthcare providers can play a critical role in identifying abuse of women with disabilities and ensuring their safety. Providers often do not ask a woman about abuse, or they may ask in front of the abuser who may be her sole caregiver.[4] Solutions to these problems may include a provider insisting that she or he consistently asks caregivers, family, and friends to leave the room during an exam. Alternatively, hospitalists may be able to fulfill this role by asking a woman if she is being abused when the woman is in the hospital after her caregiver or family and friends have left the room.

Several key indicators in the medical history may assist the healthcare professional in identifying abuse of a woman with physical disabilities. (Table 9–2). An indication of abuse may include noting a time delay between the occurrence of an injury and a subsequent visit to the doctor's office, as well as a history of the patient being "accident-prone," a history of suicide attempts, depression, multiple psychosomatic complaints, and anxiety. Other common indications to look for include panic attacks, sleep disorders, alcoholism, drug abuse, injuries during pregnancy, or symptoms of post-traumatic stress disorder (PTSD).[15-20] The physical examination of a woman's face, neck, throat, chest, breast, abdomen, and genitalia often yields indication of injuries.[15-20] McFarlane and colleagues[7] developed an abuse assessment tool sensitive to the identification of abuse in women with physical disabilities.

Intellectual Disabilities

Women with ID may respond to abuse in a manner different from that of women with physical disabilities, mainly because of their inability to clearly articulate their feelings. They may withdraw from loved ones or start acting inappropriately.[10] Additionally, they often feel negatively about themselves and have difficulty forming and maintaining relationships. It is often difficult to recognize the signs and symptoms of abuse in women with ID. Women with ID may be unable to state that they have been abused, and therefore, diagnosis requires careful observation. As scientific and anecdotal literature has shown, women with ID have "full emotional capabilities . . . [although they] may not have learned the language with which to express feelings."[10] For example, fear may be expressed through physical signs, such as incontinence or abdominal pain. It also may be expressed through behaviors like apathy, self-injury, or aggression.[10] Many times an abused woman with ID may show a decline in skills or will refuse to cooperate in tasks she used to perform. She also may begin exhibiting inappropriate sexual behavior.[10]

Table 9–2 Abuse Assessment Screen in Women with Physical Disabilities (AAS-D)

1. Within the last year, have you been hit, slapped, kicked, pushed, shoved or otherwise physically hurt by someone?   YES   NO

If yes, by who? (circle all that apply)

Intimate	Care	Health	Family	Other (e.g.,
Partner	Provider	Professional	Member	clergy, stranger)

Please describe specific relationship of abuser_____

2. Within the last year, has anyone forced you to have sexual activities?   YES   NO

If yes, who? (circle all that apply)

Intimate	Care	Health	Family	Other (e.g.,
Partner	Provider	Professional	Member	clergy, stranger)

Please describe event _____

3. Within the last year, has anyone prevented you from using a wheelchair, cane, respirator, or other assistive devices?   YES   NO

If yes, who? (circle all that apply)

Intimate	Care	Health	Family	Other (e.g.,
Partner	Provider	Professional	Member	clergy, stranger)

Please describe the episode _____

4. Within the last year, has anyone you depend on refused to help you with an important personal need, such as taking your medicine, getting to the bathroom, getting out of bed, bathing, getting dressed, or getting food or drink?   YES   NO

If yes, who? (circle all that apply)

Intimate	Care	Health	Family	Other (e.g.,
Partner	Provider	Professional	Member	clergy, stranger)

Please describe the situation_____

Source: Adapted from Nosek M, Hughes R, Taylor H, Taylor P. Disability, psychosocial, and demographic characteristics of abused women with physical disabilities. *Violence Against Women.* 2006;12(9):838–850; Petersilia J. Invisible victims: violence against persons with developmental disabilities. *Hum Rights.* 2000;27(1):9–13.

Women with ID often have PTSD that is not diagnosed because of lack of recognition of the behavioral cues.[21] Identifying whether a woman is experiencing PTSD as a result of abuse or has a behavioral problem is often difficult. A person who knows the woman well may be able to observe the behavior and identify whether this is typical for her or not. If a woman's personality is unknown, a provider may choose to perform a skills evaluation that includes evaluating problem-solving and communication skills.[10]

A thorough exam can often uncover clues to abuse. If a woman does not permit an exam initially, a provider may be able to complete the full exam through desensitization with multiple appointments. In women with communication difficulties, it is important to examine the genitals for bleeding, hematomas, or insertion of foreign objects.[10]

CLINICIAN RESPONSE TO ABUSE OF WOMEN WITH DISABILITIES

Physical Disabilities

If abuse is suspected, the healthcare provider should explain this concern to the woman and assess the degree of danger. The provider also should explain the options available to the woman and talk to her about creating a safety plan for leaving, including putting her keys, money, medications, and assistive devices in a safe place secure from the abuser. Referral to a shelter with appropriate access and services should be arranged when she is ready to leave the abuser. In 2000, the Wisconsin Coalition Against Domestic Violence published a guide for safety planning for individuals with physical disabilities. This may be given to the victim as a resource and is available at http://www.ncall.us/docs/Disability_Safety_Plan.pdf.[22] This guide helps women develop a safety plan that includes setting up alternative care providers in an acute situation.[22] Similar to all resources for women who are victims of abuse, any information provided should be very small in size and able to be hidden from the abuser. Barriers to leaving for women with physical disabilities include fear of retribution, poor health, worry about future caregiving, and lack of mobility or transportation.[16]

Physicians should aim to decrease women's vulnerability to abuse while increasing their awareness. This includes improving social and financial resources, educating the woman on how to care for herself as much as possible, and providing support and educational groups. A proposed educational program includes relationship building, communication, and stress management.[16]

Intellectual Disabilities

Although many shelters feel comfortable caring for adults with ID, they describe limitations to providing appropriate care that may be due to lack of funding. This makes it difficult to provide appropriate staffing, as well as having staff with disability-specific education.[23] If a shelter is not an option, an alternate location for a "safe house" may be required. To help facilitate the process, a provider may need to assess guardianship, financial resources, and insurance, along with transportation needs.

CONCLUSION

Abuse of women with disabilities occurs frequently. Specific risk factors for abuse among women with disabilities include dependence on others for personal care, limited mobility, and, in women with ID, limited ability to disclose the violence. Abuse in women with disabilities lasts longer and is more severe than in women in the general population. Many shelters are not easily accessible by those with various handicaps, and staff members frequently do not have the training to deal with victims who have disabilities. Clinicians should be vigilant in screening and assessing women with disabilities for any risk of abuse.

REFERENCES

1. Focht-New G, Barol B, Clements PT, Miliken TF. Persons with developmental disability exposed to interpersonal violence and crime: approaches for intervention. *Perspect Psychiatr Care.* 2008;44(2):89–98.
2. Copel LC. Partner abuse in physically disabled women: a proposed model for understanding intimate partner violence. *Perspect Psychiatr Care.* 2006;42(2):114–129.
3. Administration on Developmental Disabilities (ADD). Washington, DC: U.S. Department of Health and Human Services; 2009. Administration for Children and Families Web site. http://www.acf.hhs.gov/opa/fact_sheets/add_factsheet.html. Accessed February 2, 2010.
4. Coker AL, Smith PH, Fadden MK. Intimate partner violence and disabilities among women attending family practice clinics. *J Womens Health (Larchmt).* 2005;14(9):829–838.
5. Nosek MEA. Disability, psychosocial, and demographic characteristics of abused women with physical disabilities. *Violence Against Women.* 2006;12(9):838–850.
6. Martin SL, Ray N, Sotres-Alvarez D, et al. Physical and sexual assault of women with disabilities. *Violence Against Women.* 2006;12(9):823–837.
7. McFarlane J, Hughes RB, Nosek MA, Groff JY, Swedlend N, Dolan Mullen P. Abuse assessment screen-disability (AAS-D): measuring frequency, type, and perpetrator of abuse toward women with physical disabilities. *J Womens Health Gend Based Med.* 2001;10(9):861–866.
8. Hassouneh-Phillips D, Curry MA. Abuse of women with disabilities: state of the science. *Rehabil Counsel Bull.* 2002;45(2):96–104.
9. Stickler HL. Interaction between family violence and mental retardation. *Ment Retard.* 2001;39(6):461–471.
10. Petersilia J. Invisible victims: violence against persons with developmental disabilities. *Hum Rights.* 2000;27(1):9–13.
11. Texas Association against Sexual Assault. Sexual abuse in persons with physical disabilities. UNT Health and Wellness Center Web site. http://www.healthcenter.unt.edu/pdf/pamphlets/sexual-abuse-and-persons-with-physical-disabilities.pdf. Accessed February 2, 2010.

12. Brownbridge DA, Restock J, Hiebert-Murphy D. The high risk of IPV against Canadian women with disabilities. *Med Sci Monit.* 2008;14(5):27-32.

13. Barrett KA, O'Day B, Roche A, Carlson BL. Intimate partner violence, health status, and health care access among women with disabilities. *Womens Health Issues.* 2009;19:94-100.

14. Young ME, Nosek MA, Howland C, Chanpong G, Rintala DH. Prevalence of abuse in women with physical disabilities. *Arch Phys Med Rehab.* 1997;78 (12 Suppl 5):S34-S38.

15. Women with disabilities. Law Students for Reproductive Justice Web site. http://lsrj.org/documents/09_Women_with_Disabilities.pdf. Accessed February 2, 2010.

16. Nosek MA. *Violence Against Women with Disabilities—Final Report* [Final report of CROWD Study: Violence Against Women with Physical Disabilities]. Houston, TX: Baylor College of Medicine; 2002.

17. Nosek M, Howland C. (1998, February). *Abuse and Women with Disabilities.* Harrisburg, PA: VAWnet, a project of the National Resource Center on Domestic Violence/Pennsylvania Coalition against Domestic Violence. Violence Against Women Web site. http://www.vawnet.org. Accessed January 4, 2010.

18. Horner-Johnson W, Drum CE. Prevalence of maltreatment of people with intellectual disabilities: a review of recently published research. *Ment Retard Dev Disabil Res Rev.* 2006;12(1):57-69.

19. Nosek MA, Hughes RB. Violence against women with physical disabilities: findings from studies conducted by the Center for Research on Women with Disabilities at Baylor College of Medicine, 1992-2002. Baylor College of Medicine Web site. http://www.bcm.edu/crowd/?pmid=1409. Accessed February 2, 2010.

20. Howland MN. Women with disabilities. In: Liebschutz JM, Frayne SM, Saxe GN, eds. *Violence Against Women: A Physician's Guide to Identification and Management.* Philadelphia, PA: American College of Physicians; 2003.

21. Ryan R. Posttraumatic stress disorder in persons with developmental disabilities. *Community Ment Health J.* 1994;30(1):45-54.

22. Permission has been granted for this material to be used in the context as originally intended. This information is excerpted from *Safety Planning: A Guide for Individuals with Physical Disabilities*, published by the Wisconsin Coalition Against Domestic Violence; 2000.

23. Chang JC, Martin SL, Moracco KE, et al. Helping women with disabilities and domestic violence: strategies, limitations, and challenges of domestic violence programs. *J Womens Health.* 2003;12(7):699-708.

Chapter 10

Intimate Partner Violence in Immigrant Women

Juliet Bradley, MD

INTRODUCTION

Intimate partner violence (IPV) poses special challenges to immigrant women. Immigrant women comprise a sizable percentage of the population of the United States, and although data about the prevalence of IPV in these immigrant populations are mixed, these women have certain vulnerabilities to abuse, including limited immigrant status, limited English, limited familiarity with US laws protecting women, geographic isolation from family and support systems, and pressures from their own immigrant communities.

Research has shown that battered immigrant women are less likely to seek help from medical and legal services as well as from informal social support structures.[1] A battered immigrant woman visiting her healthcare provider for problems not directly related to her experiences of violence may come to trust this provider more than she trusts police or social service agencies. Thus, it becomes critically important for her healthcare provider to screen for IPV and to be familiar with the ways in which American laws can protect her and help her to escape an abusive relationship.

The Violence Against Women Act (VAWA) and the U-visa program help battered women overcome the special obstacles they face in trying to escape abuse; healthcare providers must be familiar with the challenges and the solutions for these women.

IMMIGRANT WOMEN IN THE UNITED STATES AND THEIR SPECIAL VULNERABILITIES

More than 12% of the US population is foreign born,[2] and immigrants comprise a growing percentage of the total US population.[3] In 2008, a record 1,046,539 persons were naturalized as US citizens. The leading countries of birth of the new citizens were Mexico, India, and the Philippines.[4] Before the 1990s, most legal immigrants were male, but, more recently, women have accounted for just over half of all legal immigrants.[5] In addition to legal immigrants, in March, 2006, the Pew Hispanic Center estimated that there were 11.5 to 12 million undocumented immigrants residing in the United States.[6]

Immigrant women, documented and undocumented, come to their new country with the hope of creating a better life for themselves and their children. Many are compelled to migrate, fleeing political repression, severe economic pressures, domestic or sexual violence, or war. The situation in the home country may be so terrible that they choose to migrate despite the risk of life-threatening travel across international borders, often without the proper documents and processing. An immigrant woman who enters the United States without proper documentation or who overstays her visa has no avenues open to convert to legal status after arrival,[7] thus increasing her vulnerability to abuse because she has to depend more on her partner.

An immigrant woman's experience in a new country is shaped by the resources with which she arrives, including money, occupation, language skills, and education. Social networks also play an important role.[8] Women who have fled desperate poverty may have very few resources to bring to their new country.

IPV is a worldwide problem, although prevalence varies from country to country. In 2005, the World Health Organization found that the proportion of women who had ever suffered physical violence by a male partner ranged from a low of 13% in Japan to a high of 61% in provincial Peru. Sexual violence was reported to be lowest among Japanese women at 6%, whereas 59% of Ethiopian women reported such violence (Figure 10–1).[9]

There are conflicting data on the prevalence of IPV among immigrant women in the United States. Immigrant women are a heterogeneous group, representing diverse cultures; these cultures have unique characteristics that affect a woman's risk for and experience of IPV. There are also inherent difficulties in conducting good research on women whose very immigration status compels them to avoid contact with researchers, who may speak an unfamiliar language or who do not understand terms like *batter* or *abuse*. A 2009 literature review by the Robert Wood Johnson Foundation found that "the relationship between immigration status or acculturation levels and the likelihood of experiencing IPV is, at best, *inconclusive*."[10]

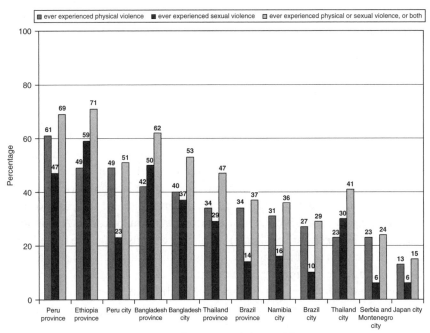

Figure 10–1 Women's experience of IPV around the world.

Source: Data from World Health Organization multi-county study on women's health and domestic violence: Initial results on prevalence, health outcomes and women's responses. Geneva, *World Health Organization*, 2005. p. 6.

Despite the comparable or even lower prevalence of IPV among immigrants, there is a higher rate of IPV-related homicide in these groups. The disproportionately high rate of homicides among immigrant groups may indicate failure and/or inadequate response to the violence by law enforcement officers and courts.[11]

Immigrant women, especially refugee women, may have experienced significant violence and/or sexual assault in their home country, in a refugee camp, or at a border crossing. This experience of violence may leave them desensitized to IPV; they may not consider the abuse by their current intimate partner to be very serious compared with the more traumatic experiences they have survived.

IPV is about power and control (see Chapter 3). Batterers classically employ various techniques to solidify this control and hamper their partners' efforts to leave the abusive relationship: isolation from the support of friends and family, enforced economic dependence on the abuser, and intimidating threats designed to prevent the woman from accessing legal and other resources.

These techniques acquire a new significance for the battered immigrant woman who might be far away from her social support system, not able to work legally, and ignorant of the laws of her new host country. Following is a discussion of some of the specific vulnerabilities immigrant women must confront.

Immigrant Status

Immigrant women who do not have the protection of US citizenship are at increased risk for IPV because of their lack of legal rights. There is a hierarchy of immigrant status: Some women are completely undocumented, some may have residency dependent on an employment visa, and others may be married to a US citizen or legal permanent resident. A woman's place in this hierarchy affects her vulnerability to abuse. Men are more likely to have the higher level immigrant status of US citizen or legal permanent resident;[12] a battered immigrant woman may be threatened by her citizen spouse with deportation or with having her children taken away from her. Her immigrant status may limit her ability to get a job and become economically independent of her abuser.

Unaware of the laws that protect her, a battered woman who is undocumented may be afraid to go to the police and afraid that if she reports the abuse she will be identified by the police as undocumented and subsequently deported. Her husband may reinforce this fear; however, Immigration and Customs Enforcement (ICE) may not begin removal proceedings against women whose undocumented status is discovered when she goes to court seeking an order of protection or child custody.[13] A refugee woman may be particularly hesitant to cause her husband's incarceration or deportation if he had been a political prisoner in his home country.

Marriage to a US citizen does not confer citizenship status. A woman whose residency status depends on her husband's petition (i.e., a woman married to a US citizen or legal permanent resident) may be threatened by her spouse that if she reports the abuse, he will not proceed with her immigration petition. Research has found that in abusive relationships, 72% of spouses who are citizens or legal permanent residents do not file immigration papers for their wives.[14] Thus, in marriages where the abuser has a higher immigrant status, a woman's residency status becomes a powerful means of control.

Immigrant women who do not depend on their marriage for their legal residency status may still be vulnerable to IPV. Legal permanent residents who come to the United States on work visas depend on their sponsored employment to remain in the country; batterers may disrupt and threaten immigrant women's jobs, jeopardizing both their employment and their ability to legally remain in the United States.

Economic Status

Many immigrants are economic refugees. They may have fled their home country because of a desperate economic situation. Arriving in the United States with limited skills and limited English precludes them from securing a well-paying job. Undocumented workers face additional challenges in the job market, including substandard pay, dangerous working conditions, and no real job security.

The economic challenges faced by the immigrant woman may make it more difficult for her to become financially independent from her abusive partner. Immigrant men who have difficulty maintaining employment are more likely to perpetrate IPV and also be more likely to have problems with substance abuse and gambling.[15]

Limited English

In addition to handicapping employment prospects, a battered woman's limited ability to speak English may pose a challenge in terms of interacting with police and with social service agencies. If the partner speaks English and the woman does not, she may have a hard time conveying her side of the story to the police. Immigrant women have often found themselves arrested because of misinformation given to the police by the batterer.[16] Limited English skills are also a barrier to obtaining appropriate social services, obtaining a certified interpreter in court, and obtaining information about their legal rights.

Importantly, the ability to speak or learn the host country's language does not always improve the situation for abused immigrant women. If an abused woman's new language abilities challenges her abuser's control and contests traditional gender roles, the abusive behavior may be exacerbated.[17]

Cultures of Origin

The cultures of origin of immigrant women may increase their vulnerability to IPV. However, immigrants hail from diverse cultures, and cultural factors relevant to Latino immigrants, for example, may not be applicable to Middle Eastern immigrants. Much of the available data about IPV in immigrant populations comes from smaller qualitative studies and testimonials and, therefore, can only be generalized in a limited way.

Cultural factors that may affect a woman's likelihood of abuse include culturally prescribed gender roles and attitudes that violence may be justified. Some cultures foster a submissive or passive role for women, whereas men gain respect for being dominant and sexually aggressive. Seventy-five percent of provincial women in the World Health Organization's 2005 study believed that violence against women is justified in some situations, commonly either female infidelity or disobedience to her husband.[18]

For many immigrant women, there is much to gain in the process of acculturation to the United States: more autonomy, more independence, more freedom. However, as women's ideologies change and they become less willing to conform to traditional gender-based roles, conflict may arise. Women entering the workforce can challenge the man's authority as a breadwinner and reduce his authority in the home. Forty-eight percent of Latinas in one study reported that their partner's violence against them had increased since they immigrated to the United States.[19]

Isolation from Family and Support System

It is common for batterers to isolate their partners from family and friends as a means of gaining control. Immigrant women may be more isolated from family and friends than US-born women whose support system is nearby. One study of south Asian immigrant women in Boston found that more than half of the sample had no family in the United States.[20]

A batterer may increase his partner's isolation by prohibiting phone calls and visits to her country of origin. He may also view acculturation to her new country as a possible challenge to his authority and thus forbid friendships with "Americans" and prohibit her from learning and speaking English and from wearing Western clothing. With family far away and the potential for development of new support networks limited by her abuser, a battered immigrant woman may feel as though she has nowhere to turn. She might feel that it is better to remain in her marriage, even if it is abusive, than to be completely isolated in a country foreign to her. And should she decide to return to her home country, she may face shame and stigma for abandoning her husband in the United States.

Limited Familiarity with US Laws Protecting Women

Many women may have emigrated from countries that do not have laws protecting women from IPV, and they may assume that US laws are similar to those in their home country. Until recently, the Mexican law called *abandono de hogar* ("abandonment of home") punished women who left their homes, even to flee violence. Women convicted of abandoning the home often lost custody of their children as well as property rights. Some Mexican women who immigrate to the United States erroneously believe that even in the United States they can be penalized under *abandono de hogar*.

Undocumented immigrants whose goal is to avoid detection by the US legal system can be intimidated by the idea of approaching that same legal system for help. They may hesitate to call the police to report abuse, past or current, worrying that they may be turned in to ICE if they interact with the criminal justice system. Advocates can remind these women that domestic violence (DV) is against the law, no matter what the legal status of the victim might be. Women should remember that they have the right to keep their immigration status private; they are not required to disclose their status to law enforcement or to shelters.[21]

Under Section 384 of the Illegal Immigration Reform and Immigrant Responsibility Act (IIRIRA), no employee of the Department of Justice (which includes ICE and immigration court personnel and judges) may "make an adverse determination" about a person's application for status "using information furnished solely by" the applicant's abuser, an abusive member of the applicant's household, or someone who has abused the applicant's child.[22]

As a matter of federal law, immigrants in all states are legally entitled to crisis counseling, police intervention, assistance from child protective services, shelter, and transitional housing for up to 2 years, treatment for mental illness or substance abuse, and other social and health assistance without having to provide verification of immigrant status.[23] Use of such resources by an immigrant woman will not affect her residency petition and may not be used as grounds to start a removal proceeding. Legal residency is *not* required to obtain an order of protection (also known as a restraining order), but orders of protection are effective only if the victim is willing to call the police to enforce the order.[24]

A batterer facing criminal prosecution because of charges brought against him by his undocumented partner may retaliate by reporting her to ICE. If she is reported, she risks being removed from the United States by ICE without being informed of her right to apply for status; ICE officials may not see educating non-citizens about their immigration rights as part of their job.

Battered women are commonly threatened with losing custody of their children. A woman's act of leaving an abusive relationship does not confer special custody rights to the father. However, if she is removed from the United States, she may lose custody of her children to her abusive legal-resident spouse. If an abusive husband threatens to take the children away or return them to his home country, the woman should apply for a custody order, which can require that the other parent not take the children out of the country or out of the state of residence. If the children are US citizens, the woman should send a copy of the custody order to the US Department of State and to the embassy of her partner's home country, as well as to the children's schools.[25]

Community Pressures

Immigrant women can be pressured by their community or religious leaders not to draw attention to the problem of IPV, believing that any community member who talks about the violence exposes the community to scorn.[26] In the current political landscape of anti-immigrant sentiment, immigrant communities may believe that issues of DV should be sorted out within the community, without involving the US legal system. This does *not* mean that DV is viewed more favorably or condoned in immigrant communities as compared with other communities; however, it does make it more difficult for service organizations to identify and assist victims.

Women who leave their abuser risk severing their connections with the larger immigrant community. This can be a very frightening prospect for immigrant women, especially those with limited English, limited economic resources, and few relationships with people outside the immigrant community. In many immigrant cultures, women who divorce their abusive spouse are blamed for breaking up their families; these divorced women are often stigmatized and ostracized from their communities.

Lack of Language-Specific or Culturally Tailored Services

Battered immigrant women may be hesitant to seek help from social service agencies if these agencies are not sensitive to their cultural concerns.[27] A DV shelter, for example, may have eating and sleeping arrangements that are very different from what the immigrant woman has known. Language and cultural differences may heighten an abused woman's sense of alienation and erode her resolve to separate from her abusive partner.

LAWS PROTECTING IMMIGRANT WOMEN

Although questions of immigration, residency status, and legal rights are best answered by an immigration lawyer, healthcare professionals who wish to advocate for patients who are victims of IPV should be familiar with the Violence Against Women Act (VAWA) and the U-visa program. In an abusive relationship, the abuser may have more physical power, more economic power, and/or more legal rights than his victim. VAWA and the U-visa program are two important means by which the US government has tried to ensure that a woman's legal status is not used as an instrument of violence and control.

Violence Against Women Act

The Violence Against Women Act (VAWA) was passed in 1994; a revision was enacted in 2000 to address various omissions and problems with implementation.[28] VAWA allows immigrant women who are legally married to US citizens or permanent legal residents to self-petition for legal residency without the knowledge or cooperation of their abusive spouse. To be eligible for VAWA, the self-petitioning spouse must[29]:

- Be legally married to the US citizen or lawful permanent resident batterer. A self-petition may be filed if the marriage was terminated by the abusive spouse's death within the 2 years before filing. A self-petition may also be filed if the marriage to the abusive spouse was terminated, within the 2 years prior to filing, by divorce related to the abuse.
- Must have been battered in the United States unless the abusive spouse is an employee of the US government or a member of the uniformed services of the United States.
- Must have been battered or subjected to extreme cruelty during the marriage or is the parent of a child who was battered or subjected to extreme cruelty by the US citizen or lawful permanent resident spouse during the marriage.
- Is required to be a person of good moral character. An act or conviction connected to the abuse will not prevent an immigration judge from finding in favor of good moral character.
- Must have entered into the marriage in good faith, not solely for the purpose of obtaining immigration benefits.

Children of the batterer can also apply for VAWA protection. Once VAWA protection is granted, a woman and her children are allowed to receive public benefits, and benefits received under VAWA may not be considered as a "public charge" in the consideration of permanent residency status. Women and children who receive VAWA protection do not have to return to their country of origin to receive their green cards when these are granted. Once VAWA protection is obtained, women are allowed to remarry before acquisition of their green card.

U-Visa and T-Visa Programs

In 2000, the Victims of Trafficking and Violence Protection Act,[30] which made improvements to the original VAWA of 1994, also created two new non-immigrant visas for non-citizen victims of crime. The U-visa and the T-visa are designed to provide immigration status to non-citizens who assist or are willing to assist authorities in the investigation of crimes. After 3 years, both U- and T-visa holders may apply for legal permanent resident status, even if the victim is not married to the abuser and even if the abuser is not a legal permanent resident.

The U-visa program offers protection to abused women who are not legally married to their partners; it is a humanitarian and material witness visa program that allows victims to obtain this temporary visa if they have suffered physical or mental injury from a crime, including IPV. The U-visa program requires that a victim has been, is being, or will be helpful in the investigation or prosecution of that crime. The T-visa program is similar to the U-visa program but is designed specifically for those who have been subjected to sex trafficking. Unlike the U-visa, applicants must show that extreme hardship involving unusual or severe harm will occur if they are removed from the United States. [31]

Political Asylum?

In the spring of 2009, government lawyers for the Department of Homeland Security stated that "it is possible . . . that applicants who have experienced domestic violence could qualify for asylum."[32] This ruling may make it possible in the future for battered immigrant women to seek asylum in the United States. At present, US law requires that applicants for asylum or refugee status must demonstrate a "well-founded fear of persecution" based on race, religion, nationality, political opinion, or "membership in a particular social group;" IPV does not fall into any of these categories. Women fleeing female genital cutting have been accepted as asylum-seekers since 1996.[33]

CONCLUSION AND IMPLICATIONS FOR THE HEALTHCARE PROVIDER

IPV is a significant human rights and public health problem worldwide (see Chapter 22), and immigrant women in the United States have special vulnerabilities to abuse. Women who have experienced violence suffer ill health compared with women who have not. Often ignorant of their rights and fearful of interacting with the US criminal justice system, an immigrant woman's encounter with her healthcare provider may offer her an opportunity to learn about her rights and ways to escape from an abusive relationship. Healthcare providers who care for battered immigrant women should be aware of the challenges they face and with the laws protecting them. Legal, medical, and social work professionals are not required to report undocumented immigrants to ICE.[34] Healthcare providers who wish to advocate for battered women should develop relationships with immigration attorneys to ensure that the women's residency status is not unwittingly jeopardized.

If an interpreter is used to obtain the patient's history, it is best to use a trained interpreter rather than family members or friends because the woman may be embarrassed to disclose abuse in their presence. Especially in smaller communities, the patient should always be asked if she knows or is related to the interpreter; doing so may help protect her privacy and help avoid further endangerment. A telephone translating service may be used if necessary. It is important to note that some immigrant women may distrust any interpreter, and the presence of any third person in the room may limit their willingness to disclose sensitive information.[35]

For specific, up-to-date legal information on IPV in immigrant women, these are some useful resources:

- www.womenslaw.org
- Family Violence Prevention Fund at http://www.endabuse.org/section/programs/immigrant_women

REFERENCES

1. Raj A, Silverman J. Violence against immigrant women: the roles of culture, context, and legal immigrant status on intimate partner violence. *Violence Against Women.* 2002;8(3):367–398.
2. Lee J, Rytina N. Naturalizations in the United States: 2008. Department of Homeland Security Web site. http://www.dhs.gov/xlibrary/assets/statistics/publications/natz_fr_2008.pdf. Accessed December 1, 2009.
3. Foreign-born population and foreign born as percentage of the total US population, 1850 to 2008. Migration Policy Institute Web site. http://www.migrationinformation.org/datahub/charts/final.fb.shtml. Accessed December 1, 2009.
4. See reference 2.
5. *The New Americans: Economic, Demographic, and Fiscal Effects of Immigration* (1997). National Academies Press Web site. http://books.nap.edu/openbook.php?record_id=5779&page=52. Accessed December 1, 2009.
6. Passel JS. The size and characteristics of the unauthorized migrant population in the US [research report, March 7, 2006]. Pew Hispanic Center Web site. http://www.pewtrusts.org/uploadedFiles/wwwpewtrustsorg/Reports/Hispanics_in_America/PHC_Immigration_0306.pdf. Accessed December 1, 2009.

7. Intimate partner violence in immigrant and refugee communities: challenges, promising practices and recommendations (report by the Family Violence Prevention Fund for the Robert Wood Johnson Foundation, March 2009). Robert Wood Johnson Web site. http://www.rwjf.org/files/research/ipvreport 20090331.pdf

8. Menjivar C, Salcido O. Immigrant women and domestic violence: common experiences in different countries. *Gender Soc.* 2002;16(6):898–920.

9. World Health Organization. *Multi-County Study on Women's Health and Domestic Violence: Initial Results on Prevalence, Health Outcomes and Women's Responses.* Geneva, Switzerland: World Health Organization; 2005:6.

10. See reference 7.

11. See reference 7.

12. See reference 1.

13. Womens Law.org Web site. http://www.womenslaw.org. Accessed August 29, 2009.

14. See reference 1.

15. Morash M, Bui M, Santiago A. Gender specific ideology of domestic violence in Mexican origin families. *Int Rev Victimology.* 2000;7:67–91.

16. See reference 7.

17. See reference 8.

18. See reference 9.

19. Dutton M, Orloff L, Aguilar Hass G. Characteristics of help-seeking behaviors, resources, and services needs of battered Latina immigrants: legal and policy implications. *Georgetown J Poverty Law Policy.* 2000;7(2):245–301.

20. See reference 1.

21. Immigration: basic questions & answers. WomensLaw.org Web site. http://www. womenslaw.org/laws_state_type.php?id=10269&state_code=US&open_id=1083 2#content-10832. Accessed December 31, 2009.

22. Illegal Immigration Reform and Responsibility Act of 1996, Division C of the Omnibus Appropriations Act of 1996 (H.R. 3610), Pub. L. No. 104-208, 110 Stat. 3009.

23. See reference 1.

24. Immigration: basic questions & answers. WomensLaw.org Web site. http://www. womenslaw.org/laws_state_type.php?id=10269&state_code=US#content-10815. Accessed December 31, 2009.

25. Immigration: basic questions & answers. WomensLaw.org Web site. http://www. womenslaw.org/laws_state_type.php?id=10269&state_code=US#content-10816. Accessed January 11, 2010.

26. See reference 7.

27. Orloff LE, Little R. *Somewhere to Turn: Making Domestic Violence Services Available to Battered Immigrant Women. A "How-To" Manual for Battered Women's Advocates and Service Providers.* Washington, DC: Ayuda Inc; 1999.

28. Excerpts from the Victims of Trafficking and Violence Protection Act of 2000 (VAWA 2000). US Department of Justice Web site. http://www.ovw.usdoj.gov/ laws/vawo2000/welcome.html. Accessed January 11, 2010.

29. US Citizenship and Immigration Services Web site. http://www.uscis.gov/portal/ site/uscis/menuitem. Accessed December 31, 2009.

30. 114 Stat. 1464, Pub. L. 106-386 (Oct. 28, 2000).
31. Victims of Trafficking Act, §§ 103(8) & (9).
32. Door opens for battered immigrant women seeking asylum. Family Violence Prevention Fund Web site. http://www.endabuse.org/content/features/detail/1316/. Accessed November 7, 2009.
33. Kim Y. CRS report for Congress: Asylum law and female genital mutilation: recent developments. Order Code RS22810. February 2008. Federation of American Scientists Web site. http://www.fas.org/sgp/crs/misc/RS22810.pdf. Accessed December 31, 2009.
34. See reference 28.
35. Julliard K, Vivar J, Delgado C, Cruz E, Kabak J, Sabers H. What Latina patients don't tell their doctors: a qualitative study. *Ann Fam Med.* 2008;6(6):543-549.

Chapter 11

Intimate Partner Violence in Pregnancy

Rose S. Fife, MD, MPH

INTRODUCTION

During pregnancy, women are at increased risk of intimate partner violence (IPV).[1,2] This occurs most commonly in a relationship in which some type of IPV (not necessarily physical) already occurs.[2,3] The violence may change from verbal or psychological abuse to physical or sexual abuse during pregnancy because of the stress of the pregnancy itself on the relationship, especially if both partners did not want the pregnancy equally.[2] However, for some couples pregnancy is the first time that any abuse occurs.[3] There are several theories for this increase in violence. Many relate to the idea of power and control as the central tenet of an abusive relationship (see Chapters 2 and 6).[2,4-7] Among couples in which the woman is already being abused, the pregnancy may make the male partner feel less in control because of the presence of a fetus, which he may view as a rival.[2,4-7] Pregnancy, especially in the third trimester, may make sexual intercourse more challenging, which also may anger the man.[2,4-7] In couples who have not previously had an abusive relationship, pregnancy also may represent a challenge to a man who thinks he is in control, even without abuse; it may be the "last straw" that drives him to abusive behavior.[2,4-7]

Cultural norms are likely to affect the occurrence of IPV during pregnancy.[3] As noted in many of the other chapters in this book (Chapters 6 and 10), acceptance of abuse by women differs among cultures, with more acceptance of gender inequity among African Americans, Latinos, and other groups.[7]

STATISTICS

It has been estimated that as many as 20% of all pregnancies may be complicated by various forms of IPV.[8] According to the Bureau of Justice Statistics,[9] IPV in pregnancy accounts for approximately 6% of all IPV among women older than 18 years in the United States each year. IPV is the leading cause of maternal mortality and adverse maternal outcomes in the United States.[1,2,10,11] IPV during pregnancy is associated with increased chances of low birthweight or preterm babies.[12]

As is true for all types of family violence, IPV in pregnancy crosses all socioeconomic groups.[8,13-15] IPV during pregnancy also is more common among teens than adults.[16,17]

CAUSES/RISK FACTORS

Again, as is true for other forms of family violence, women who have suffered from or witnessed abuse at other times in their lives are more likely to be victims of IPV during pregnancy.[1,10] Use of alcohol or drugs also increases the risk of IPV during pregnancy, as in other stages of life.[1,18,19] As many as 45% of males and 20% of females have been reported to be drinking at the time of abuse.[19]

INTERVENTIONS

Screening for abuse is strongly advocated by the American Congress of Obstetricians and Gynecology (ACOG)[2,20] and others[21-24] during all trimesters of pregnancy. Shockingly, one study indicated that healthcare providers actually saw approximately 47% of all victims who were murdered or were victims of attempted murder in the context of IPV during the year before they died.[2,25] Several screening tools are available, including a very brief (2-minute) Abuse Assessment Screen.[26,27] Rodriguez et al[28] found that about two-thirds of a group of Latinas in Los Angeles had never been screened for IPV during pregnancy, and they developed a questionnaire that was then pilot-tested. The results indicated that having a simple test that was readily available to healthcare providers could improve the frequency of testing. Interestingly, a prospective observational study regarding the willingness of pregnant women to answer screening questions was inversely associated with their IPV experience during pregnancy.[29] The authors speculated that the victims were afraid of increased abuse if they revealed any information.

As noted elsewhere, the three levels of prevention are primary, secondary, and tertiary.[30,31] In the case of pregnancy,[13] primary prevention would involve interventions before any abuse has occurred. Secondary prevention would involve intervening at an early stage. Tertiary prevention would include caring for women who have suffered serious IPV during pregnancy.

The Stages of Change Transtheoretical Model (TTM), described by DiClemente and Prochaska,[32,33] has been used as the basis of some interventions designed to reduce IPV during pregnancy. It is based on the concept that an individual's willingness to alter his or her behavior occurs through a sequence of stages, from lack of awareness of the problem to taking major action to change one's situation and then maintaining the new status. The various interventions range from providing information about IPV and pregnancy to those who do not recognize any problem all the way through safety planning and essentially starting a new life.[2] A community-wide primary care research study, DC-HOPE, has been developed for African American women in Washington, D.C., to improve all pregnancy outcomes, including reduction of IPV.[15] The program consists of 10 sessions that covered a variety of areas of concern, including smoking, depression, and IPV, which were all considered adverse risk factors for pregnancy outcomes. Follow-up indicated that this behavioral intervention decreased the psychosocial risk factors related to IPV.[34]

Another community-based intervention (MOSAIC: MOther's Advocates in the Community) is being piloted in Melbourne, Australia, to compare a control arm with a "treatment" group in which "disadvantaged" women who were pregnant or postpartum receive 12 months of support from "mentor mothers."[35]

SUMMARY

IPV in pregnancy spans all socioeconomic groups and is one of the leading causes of maternal morbidity and mortality, as well as adverse outcomes of pregnancy. It is underreported and underrecognized like all other forms of family violence. Obstetric providers have a unique opportunity to intercede and have certainly stepped up to deal with this condition to a great extent. Nonetheless, much more needs to be done by society and the healthcare professions.

Issues of safety for mother and baby must be addressed in the setting of IPV during and after pregnancy. Not only should physicians and nurses be mindful of the multiple serious outcomes of trauma to both mother and infant, but plans should be made for the safe removal of the mother and baby from the violent home when the mother is ready to leave.

REFERENCES

1. Chambliss LR. Intimate partner violence and its implication for pregnancy. *Clin Obstet Gynecol.* 2008;51:385–397.
2. Kramer A. Stages of change: surviving IPV during and after pregnancy. *J Perinat Neonat Nurs.* 2007;21:285–295.
3. Ellsberg M. Violence against women and the Millennium Development Goals: facilitating women's access to support. *Int J Gynecol Obstet.* 2006;94:325–332.
4. Humphrey J, Campbell JC, eds. *Family Violence and Nursing Practice.* Philadelphia, PA: Lippincott Williams and Wilkins; 2003.
5. Campbell J, Rose L, Kub J, Nedd D. Voices of strength and resistance: a contextual and longitudinal analysis of women responses to battering. *J Interpers Violence.* 1998;13:743–761.
6. Campbell JC, Oliver CE, Bullock LF. The dynamics of battering during pregnancy: Women's explanations of why. In: Campbell JC, ed. *Empowering Survivors of Abuse: Healthcare for Battered Women and Their Children.* Thousand Oaks, CA: Sage; 1998:81–89.
7. Matteson S, Rodriguez E. Battering in pregnant Latinas. *Issues Ment Health Nurs.* 1999;20:405–422.
8. Bailey BA, Daugherty RA. Intimate partner violence during pregnancy: incidence and associated health behaviors in a rural population. *Matern Child Health J.* 2007;11:495–503.
9. Bureau of Justice Statistics. Criminal victimization in the U.S., 1998 Statistical Tables. NCJ 2000 (181585).
10. Goodman PE. The relationship between intimate partner violence and other forms of family and societal violence. *Emerg Med Clin N Am.* 2006;24:889–903.
11. Plichta SB. IPV and physical health consequences. Policy and practice implications. *J Interpers Violence.* 2004;19:1296–1323.
12. Wilkinson DS, Korenbrot CC, Greene J. A performance indicator of psychosocial services in enhanced prenatal care of Medicaid eligible women. *Matern Child Health J.* 1998;2:131–143.
13. Shoffner DH. We don't like to think about it: IPV during pregnancy and postpartum. *J Perinat Neonat Nurs.* 2008;22:39–48.
14. Rodriguez MA, Heilemann MV, Fielder E, Ang A, Nevarez F, Mangione CM. Intimate partner violence, depression, and PTSD among pregnant Latina women. *Ann Fam Med.* 2008;6(1):44–52.
15. Katz KS, Blake SM, Milligan RA, et al. The design, implementation and acceptability of an integrated intervention to address multiple behavioral and psychosocial risk factors among pregnant African American women. *BMC Pregnancy Childbirth.* 2008;8:1–22.
16. Glass N, et al. Adolescent dating violence: prevalence, risk factors, health outcomes, and implications for clinical practice. *J Obstet Gynecol Neonatal Nurs.* 2003;32:227–238.
17. Tan LH, Quinlivan JA. Domestic violence, single parenthood, and fathers in the setting of teenage pregnancy. *J Adolesc Health.* 2006;38:201–207.
18. New perspectives in alcohol's role in marital violence. Journal Watch Web site. http://www.psychiatry.jwatch.org. Accessed November 23, 2009.

19. Kyriacou DN, Anglin D, Taliaferro E, et al. Risk factors for injury to women from domestic violence against women. *N Engl J Med*. 1999;34(25):1892–1898.
20. American Congress of Obstetricians and Gynecologists. IPV and domestic violence. In special issues of *Women's Health*. Washington, DC. 2005;AC06:169–188.
21. Calderon SH, Gilbert P, Jackson R, Kohn MA, Gerbert B. Cueing prenatal providers: effects on discussions of intimate partner violence. *Am J Prev Med*. 2008;34:134–137.
22. Duncan MM, McIntosh PA, Stayton CD, Hall CB. Individualized performance feedback to increase prenatal domestic violence screening. *Matern Child Health J*. 2006;10:443–449.
23. Renker PR, Tonkin P. Postpartum women's evaluations of an audio/video computer-assisted perinatal violence screen. *Comput Inform Nurs*. 2006;25:139–147.
24. Jeanjot I, Barlow P, Rozenberg S. Domestic violence during pregnancy: survey of patients and healthcare providers. *J Womens Health*. 2008;17:557–567.
25. Parsons L, Goodwin MM, Petersen R. Violence against women and reproductive health: toward defining a role for reproductive health care services. *Matern Child Health J*. 2000;4:135–140.
26. McFarlane J, Parker B, Soeken K, Bullock L. Assessing for abuse during pregnancy: severity and frequency of injuries and associated entry into prenatal care. *JAMA*. 1992;267:3176–3178.
27. McFarlane J, Parker B, Soeken K, Silva C, Reel S. Safety behaviors of abused women after an intervention during pregnancy. *J Obstet Gynecol Neonat Nurs*. 1998;27:64–69.
28. Rodriguez M, Shoultz J, Richardson E. Intimate partner screening and pregnant Latinas. *Violence Vict*. 2009;24:520–532.
29. Yost NP, Bloom SL, McIntire DD, Leveno KJ. A prospective observational study of domestic violence during pregnancy. *Obstet Gynecol*. 2005;106:61–65.
30. Gordon RS. An operational classification of disease prevention. *Public Health Rep*. 1983;98(2):107–109.
31. Walker HM, Shinn MR. Structuring school-based interventions to achieve integrated primary, secondary, and tertiary prevention goals for safe and effective schools. In: Shinn M, Walker HM, Stoner G, eds. *Interventions for Academic and Behavior Problems II: Preventive and Remedial Approaches*. Bethesda, MD: NASP Publications; 2002:1–25.
32. Prochaska J, DiClemente CC, Norcross J. In search of how people change: application to addictive behaviors. *Am Psychol*. 1992;47:1102–1114.
33. DiClemente CC, Prochaska JO. Toward a comprehensive, transtheoretical model of change: stages of change and addictive behaviors. In: Miller WR, Healther N, eds. *Treating Addictive Behaviors*. 2nd ed. New York: Plenum; 1998:3–24.
34. Joseph JG, El-Mohandes AA, Kiely M, et al. Reducing psychosocial and behavioral pregnancy risk factors: results of a randomized clinical trial among high-risk pregnant African American women. *Am J Public Health*. 2009;99:1053–1061.
35. Taft AJ, Small R, Hegarty KL, Lumley J, Watson LF, Gold L. MOSAIC (MOtherS' Advocates In the Community): protocol and sample description of a cluster randomized trial of mentor mother support to reduce IPV among pregnant or recent mothers. *BMC Public Health*. 2009;9:159.

Chapter 12

Dating Violence in Adolescents

Rose S. Fife, MD, MPH

INTRODUCTION

Teen dating violence (TDV) can be defined as intimate partner abuse (emotional, psychological, physical, sexual) in an adolescent dating relationship.[1] Unlike intimate partner violence (IPV) in adults and dating violence in older teens, violence among younger teens tends to be more equally divided between females and males.[2] The younger the individuals, the more likely it is that the girls are the perpetrators.[2,3] However, violence among younger teens tends to be verbal (e.g., name-calling, insults), psychological (e.g., bullying, spreading falsehoods),[2] or physical (e.g., hitting, slapping), which is different from what is encountered among older teens when male abuse of females is more common and includes the additional components of sexual aggression and greater physical abuse.[4,5] The reason for this change in pattern and gender prevalence with age is not well understood. However, in some cases the violence perpetrated by the female represents a defensive reaction to abusive behaviors of the male.[6,7]

Adolescents may not have a good grounding in what so-called healthy or respectful relationships mean. Their models may be based on abusive home environments because TDV tends to be more common among those living in such households, whether because of abuse to themselves as children[8-10] or an abusive parental relationship.[11] Several studies have shown that they may be more influenced by the behaviors of their peers than by their parents, so that if their friends are in abusive relationships, they are at greater risk for the same.[9-13] Thus, they may have misconceptions about a "normal" relationship based on the examples in their environment. Young people are usually not skilled in negotiations, so they may not be able to thwart abusive or otherwise uncomfortable relationships or unwanted advances.[9] They also typically do not seek help if they find themselves in such a relationship.[14]

STATISTICS

Numbers are very useful in understanding any form of abuse. However, very large ranges of incidence and prevalence for TDV have been reported in the literature, which is consistent with inaccurate reporting.[15] As is true for all other forms of IPV, TDV is under-reported.[3] The 2005 Youth Risk Behavior Surveillance System (YRBSS) reported that 9.2% of teens said that they had been victims of TDV, a number that has apparently been stable since 1999.[16-18] According to the National Coalition Against Domestic Violence (NCADV),[3] adolescent women are victims of at least 38% of all date rapes in the United States each year. Furthermore, women between the ages of 16 and 24 years have the highest per capita rate of IPV at 16%, compared with 6% for all women.[3] As an aside, it should be noted that this 6% rate of IPV is much lower than the usual reported rates in the literature. Approximately a third of teens report that someone they know has suffered from date rape.[3]

In one study, 25% of female adolescents reported physical or sexual abuse during a date.[19] In another study, over a third reported being victims of dating violence.[20] In a third study, 9.5% of all females in grades 7–12 reported ever perpetrating physical violence in a dating setting, and 6.1% reported ever perpetrating sexual abuse.[6] Adolescents who have been subjected to TDV are at higher risk for IPV as they get older.[20-22]

CAUSES OF TEEN DATING VIOLENCE (RISK FACTORS)

Why do young people harm each other in dating relationships? There are numerous theories. One involves the teen's own personal history of child abuse or witnessing other forms of family violence in their own homes.[5,9,11] Exposure to such violence seems to play a significant role in future abuse or victimization.[21,22] Cultural attitudes and behaviors often are important, too.[23] In some groups, males are considered stronger, wiser, superior to females, and thus have the "right" to treat women however they choose.[6,9,13,21,24-26] In some groups, the concept that women are not supposed to object to any abuse but accept it as their "duty" prevails.[24] Greater acceptance of stereotyping by gender has been noted among some minority teens, especially African

Americans and Latinos.[24] However, as noted earlier, several studies have indicated that peer influence on teens may be the most important factor in their attitudes toward abusive behaviors.[6,10,11]

Teens whose peer group includes abuse tend to experience higher rates of TDV than other teens.[10,11] In some studies, the behavioral norms of the peer group outweigh even familial influences.[10,11] As noted earlier, a very substantial number of teens know a peer who has been abused.

Risk factors for TDV have been reported to include those coming from single-parent homes, living in rural areas, being members of minority groups,[24] having little parental supervision, having a history of being abused as a child or witnessing abuse at home, belief structures (e.g., violence is "okay"), substance abuse (drug and/or alcohol), practicing risky sex, having peers who condone violent behavior or have a history of TDV themselves, and dropping out of school.[25,27-30] However, as in IPV, all socioeconomic groups are affected by TDV.[24]

An individual's self-esteem likely plays some role in being the victim of dating abuse.[5,9] Adolescence is a period during which teens try to learn who they are and where they are going. These goals are obviously affected by how they see themselves. A teen who has grown up in a family or who belongs to a peer group in which she or he is constantly insulted, put down, ignored, and so on, is likely to think that she or he is not worth much and may be more willing to do whatever it takes to become a part of a group, whether that is a collection of friends or a romantic dyad. If the "significant other" abuses her or him, she or he may well be more likely to tolerate it than a teen who has a good sense of self-worth.[8,11,21]

CONSEQUENCES OF TEEN DATING VIOLENCE

As is true for all forms of intimate partner abuse, TDV is associated with poor health and mental consequences. Numerous studies have found associations between TDV and a variety of unhealthy outcomes, such as smoking, consuming alcohol, being depressed or suicidal, and overeating.[19,30-32] In addition, teens who are the victims of rape as part of dating violence are at much greater risk of acquiring sexually transmitted diseases, including HIV/AIDS, or becoming pregnant, because they are unlikely to be able to negotiate the use of condoms and other protective devices.[13,30]

INTERVENTION AND PREVENTION

Some researchers have called for screening and recognition as a first step in reducing or preventing TDV. Brown et al[33] conducted an Internet study of psychiatrists and found that they did not screen consistently for IPV.

Glass and colleagues[30] reviewed routine screening practices reported in the literature and suggested that offering teens the opportunity to respond to questions about IPV in the relatively safe setting of a healthcare provider's office encouraged them to talk about their experience with TDV. A variety of advocacy groups, from professional organizations to nonprofits, have called for routine screening for TDV (and IPV).[30] Rickert et al[9] have recommended that screening tools be used to measure victimization and attitudes associated with TDV. Several specific screening tools have been developed to assess risks for TDV, including the widely used Conflict in Adolescent Dating Relationships Inventory (CADRI).[34]

Three types of prevention, regardless of the condition under study, are commonly described (1) primary, which is targeted at preventing the occurrence of a disorder or condition in the first place; (2) secondary, which aims to reduce harm from exposure to the condition; and (3) tertiary, which targets those who have had substantial exposure.[35] These concepts arise from the original approach to prevention of diseases, in which primary prevention protected the individual from getting the disease, secondary prevention represented early treatment, and tertiary occurred after the establishment of a chronic disease or disability to keep the condition from making the individual even sicker.[36]

Several approaches have been developed over the years as intervention attempts for TDV. A few are discussed here. Many programs are based in schools. A Task Force on Community Preventive Services convened by the Centers for Disease Control and Prevention (CDC) conducted a systematic review of the literature on the subject, and 56 studies of universal school-based programs were identified that met their criteria for review.[37] This report of the effectiveness of such school-based interventions was released by the CDC in 2007.[37] Its findings led to the Task Force's recommendation for "the use of universal school-based programs to prevent or reduce violent behavior" (including TDV).

Safe Dates, created by Foshee and colleagues,[38–40] is a 9- to 10-week school-based program that includes a curriculum, presentation of plays by the students, poster contests, community services for teens involved in TDV, and educational programs for community providers. The goals of the program include changing teen behaviors and increasing their ability to resolve conflicts. It has been evaluated by its developers over the years. In the initial 1-year follow-up, short-term behavioral modifications had disappeared, but effects on attitudes regarding dating violence norms, the ability to manage conflicts, and the ability to access community services for help persisted.[38] At the 4-year follow-up,[40] those participating in the program reported statistically significantly less violence in dating relationships than did those in the control (i.e., those not participating in the program) group. "Booster" sessions of the program did not affect the results. Because Safe Dates was developed for a rural population, its generalizability has not been established. However, it is commonly used around the country because of its ease and the lack of many alternatives.

The "Expect Respect" program was developed in 1988 and targets building teen self-esteem and respect for others.[41] It includes adoption of school policies regarding violence, activities to make students and families aware of the problem of TDV, leadership training for teens, and support groups at schools for teens who are "at risk" or have experienced TDV. A qualitative evaluation was reported in 2009[41] and suggested that the support groups were particularly useful for teens. Recommendations also emerged regarding the importance of respect for others, "positive relationships," and skill building. The program has so far been conducted only in schools in Austin, Texas, and thus its generalizability also is not known.

DATING VIOLENCE AND RAPE IN COLLEGE STUDENTS

College-age students are in a category of their own, considered neither adolescents nor adults. Thus, we feel that a separate section is warranted on this group and their issues.

As noted earlier, as teens age, IPV tends to occur along the lines it does in adults (more male aggression against females) than what is seen in young teens (more female aggression). College is a stage in life at which teens are, to a very large extent, on their own, in many cases both away from their families and their former peer group. Dating violence in teens includes the same types of abuse as in other groups: psychological, physical, sexual, and financial. Control is the underlying motivation as is true in other age groups. One study reported that in a 1-year period, 15.4% of college women had experienced an episode that met the legal definition of rape, and another 12.1% reported an attempted rape.[42,43] Dating violence is probably as underreported, if not more so, than any other form of IPV.

Follingstad and colleagues[44] have found that issues of control and anger are associated with dating violence and rape in college students. Several authors have shown that exposure to violence in one's own family affected college students' susceptibility to IPV just as it does in adolescents and adults.[45-48]

The use of drugs and ethanol has been associated with college dating violence and rape, as it has with IPV in adults and older adolescents.[49-51] It should always be pointed out that these agents do not cause abuse or rape, but they can lead to greater aggression in some already aggressive individuals, and they also can reduce one's inhibitions and make unsafe practices seem less unsafe.

Several interventions for college dating violence and rape have been described and implemented.[42,52–56] Some of these include the annual "Take Back the Night" rally and march on many college campuses that seeks to raise awareness and offer support to college students.[53] Another program used on college campuses is called "A Long Walk Home."[54] Some acting groups travel to various colleges to perform skits and lead discussions.[55] Another group, Prevention Connection, has Web-based programs to prevent dating violence and rape targeting college students.[56] A recent article discussed the "proliferation" of rape prevention programs, pointing out that most of their outcomes remained unknown.[57]

REFERENCES

1. National Youth Violence Prevention Resource Center. Teen Dating Violence. STYRVE Web site. http://www.safeyouth.org/scripts/index.asp. Accessed November 22, 2009.
2. Fredland NM. Sexual bullying: addressing the gap between bullying and dating violence. *Adv Nurs Sci.* 2008;31:95–105.
3. Dating violence facts. National Coalition Against Domestic Violence Web site. http://ncadv.org/. Accessed November 22, 2009.
4. Wekerle C, Wolfe DA. Dating violence in mid-adolescence: Theory, significance, and emerging prevention initiatives. *Clin Psychol Rev.* 1999;19:435–456.
5. Wolfe DA, Wekerle C, Scott K, Straatman Al, Graskey C. Predicting abuse in adolescent dating relationships over 1 year: the role of child maltreatment and trauma. *J Abnorm Psychol.* 2004;113:406–415.
6. Banyard VL, Cross C, Modecki KL. Interpersonal violence in adolescence: ecological correlates of self-reported perpetration. *J Interpers Violence.* 2006;21:1314–1332.
7. Foshee VA, Bauman KE, Linder F, Rice J, Wilcher R. Typologies of adolescent dating violence: identifying typologies of adolescent dating violence perpetration. *J Interpers Violence.* 2007;22:498–519.
8. Gagne M-H, Lavoie F, Hebert M. Victimization during childhood and revictimization in dating relationships in adolescent girls. *Child Abuse Negl.* 2005;29:1155–1172.
9. Rickert VI, Vaughan RD, Weimann CM. Adolescent dating violence and date rape. *Curr Opin Obstet Gynecol.* 2002;14:495–500.
10. Bossarte RM, Simon TR, Swahn MH. Clustering of adolescent dating violence, peer violence, and suicidal behavior. *J Interpers Violence.* 2008;23:815–833.
11. Arriaga XB, Foshee VA. Adolescent dating violence: do adolescents follow in their friends', or their parents', footsteps? *J Interpers Violence.* 2004;19:162–184.
12. Levendosky AA, Huth-Bocks A, Semel MA. Adolescent peer relationships and mental health functioning in families with domestic violence. *J Clin Child Psychol.* 2002;31:206–218.

13. Sears HA, Byers ES, Whelan JJ, Saint-Pierre M. "If it hurts you, then it is not a joke": adolescents' ideas about girls' and boys' use and experience of abusive behavior in dating relationships. *J Interpers Violence*. 2006;21:1191-1207.

14. Ashley OS, Foshee VA. Adolescent help-seeking for dating violence: prevalence, sociodemographic correlates, and sources of help. *J Adolesc Health*. 2005;36:25-31.

15. Betz CL. Teen dating violence: an unrecognized health care need [editorial]. *J Pediatr Nurs*. 2007;22:427-429.

16. YRBS—Selected Steps Communities, 2005. *MMWR Wkly Rep*. 2007;56 (SS-2):1-16.

17. Grunbaum JA, Kann L, Kinchen S, et al. Youth risk behavior surveillance—United States, 2003. *MMWR Surveill Summ*. 2004;53(SS-2):1-98.

18. Centers for Disease Control and Prevention. Physical dating violence among high school students—United States, 2003. *MMWR Morb Mortal Wkly Rep*. 2006; 55:532-535.

19. Silverman J G, Raj A, Mucci LA, Hathaway JE. Dating violence against adolescent girls and associated substance use, unhealthy weight control, sexual risk behavior, pregnancy, and suicidality. *JAMA*. 2001;286:572-579.

20. Forcier M, Patel R, Kahn JA. Pediatric residents' attitudes and practices regarding adolescent dating violence. *Ambul Pediatr*. 2003;3:317-323.

21. Taylor CA, Sorenson SB. Injunctive social norms of adults regarding teen dating violence. *J Adolesc Health*. 2004;34:468-479.

22. Smith PH, White JH, Holland IJ. A longitudinal perspective on dating violence among adolescent and college-age women. *Am J Public Health*. 2003;93:1104-1109.

23. Ulloa EC, Jaycox LH, Marshall GN, Collings RL. Acculturation, gender stereotypes, and attitudes about dating violence among Latino youth. *Violence Vict*. 2004;19:273-287.

24. Foshee VA, Karriker-Jaffe KJ, Reyes HL, et al. What accounts for demographic differences in trajectories of adolescent dating violence? An examination of intrapersonal and contextual mediators. *J Adolesc Health*. 2008;42:596-604.

25. Spencer GA, Bryant SA. Dating violence: a comparison of rural, suburban, and urban teens. *J Adolesc Health*. 2000;27:302-305.

26. Foshee VA, Linder F, MacDougall JE, Bangdiwala S. Gender differences in the longitudinal predictors of adolescent dating violence. *Prevent Med*. 2001;32:128-141.

27. St. Mars T, Valdez AM. Adolescent dating violence: understanding what is "at risk?"' *J Emerg Nurs*. 2007;33:492-494.

28. Vezina J, Hebert M. Risk factors for victimization in romantic relationships of young women. *Trauma Violence Abuse*. 2007;8:33-66.

29. Roudsari BS, Leahy MM, Walters ST. Correlates of dating violence among male and female heavy-drinking college students. *J Interpers Violence*. 2009;24:1892-1905.

30. Glass N, Friedland N, Campbell J, Yonas M, Sharps P, Kub J. Adolescent dating violence: prevalence, risk factors, health outcomes, and implications for clinical practice. *J Obstet Gynecol Neonatal Nurs*. 2003;32:227-238.

31. Ackard DM, Eisenberg ME, Neumark-Sztainer D. Long-term impact of adolescent dating violence on the behavioral and psychological health of male and female youth. *J Pediatr*. 2007;151:476-481.

32. Banyard VL, Cross C. Consequences of teen dating violence: understanding intervening variables in ecological context. *Violence Against Women*. 2008;14:998-1013.

33. Brown LK, Puster KL, Vazquez EA, Hunter HL, Lescano CM. Screening practices for adolescent dating violence. *J Interpers Violence.* 2007;22:456–464.

34. Wolfe DA, Scott K, Reitzel-Jaffe D, et al. Development and validation of the conflict in adolescent dating relationship inventory. *Psychol Assess.* 2001;13:277–293.

35. Gordon RS Jr. An operational classification of disease prevention. *Public Health Rep.* 1983;98:107–109.

36. Walker HM, Shinn MR. Structuring school-based interventions to achieve integrated primary, secondary, and tertiary prevention goals for safe and effective schools. In: Shinn M, Walker HM, Stoner G, eds. *Interventions for Academic and Behavior Problems II: Preventive and Remedial Approaches.* Bethesda, MD: NASP Publications; 2002:1–25.

37. Task Force on Community Preventive Services, CDC. The effectiveness of universal school-based programs for the prevention of violent and aggressive behavior. *MMWR Morb Mortal Wkly Rep.* 2007;56(No. RR-7):1–6.

38. Foshee VA, Bauman KE, Arriaga XB, Helms RW, Koch GG, Linder GF. An evaluation of Safe Dates, an adolescent dating violence prevention program. *Am J Public Health.* 1998;88:45–50.

39. Foshee VA, Bauman KE, Greene WF, Koch FF, Linder GF, MacDougall JE. The Safe Dates program: 1-year follow-up results. *Am J Public Health.* 2000;90:1619–1622.

40. Foshee VA, Bauman KE, Ennet ST, Linder GF, Benefield T, Suchindran C. Assessing the long-term effects of the Safe Dates Program and a booster in preventing and reducing adolescent dating violence victimization and perpetration. *Am J Public Health.* 2004;94:619–624.

41. Ball B, Kerig PK, Rosenbluth B. Like a family but better because you can actually trust each other: The Expect Respect Dating Violence Prevention Program for at-risk youth. *Health Promot Pract.* 2009;10:45S–58S.

42. Lanier CA, Elliott MN, Martin DW, Kapadia A. Evaluation of an intervention to change attitudes toward date rape. *J Am Col Health.* 1998;46:177–180.

43. Follingstad DR, Bradley RG, Laughlin JE, Burke L. Risk factors and correlates of dating violence: the relevance of examining frequency and severity levels in a college sample. *Violence Vict.* 1999;14:365–380.

44. Follingstad DR, Bradley RG, Helff CM, Laughlin JE. A model for predicting dating violence: anxious attachment, angry temperament, and need for relationship control. *Violence Vict.* 2002;17:35–47.

45. Gover AR, Kaukinen C, Fox KA. The relationship between violence in the family of origin and dating violence among college students. *J Interpers Violence.* 2008;23:1667–1693.

46. Kaura SA, Allen CM. Dissatisfaction with relationship power and dating violence perpetration by men and women. *J Interpers Violence.* 2004;19:576–588.

47. Koss P, Gidycz CA, Wisniewski N. The scope of rape: incidence and prevalence of sexual aggression and victimization in a national sample of higher education students. *J Consult Clin Psychol.* 1987;55:162–170.

48. Noland VJ, Liller KD, McDermott RJ, Coulter ML, Seraphine AE. Is adolescent sibling violence a precursor to college dating violence? *Am J Health Behav.* 2004;28(Suppl 1):S13–S23.

49. Crawford E, Wright MO, Birchmeier Z. Drug-facilitated sexual assault: college women's perception and behavioral choices. *J Am Coll Health.* 2008;57:261–272.

50. Mohler-Juo M, Dowdall GW, Koss MP, Wechsler H. Correlates of rape while intoxicated in a national sample of college women. *J Stud Alcohol.* 2004;65:37–45.

51. Young A, Grey M, Abbey A, Boyd CJ, McCabe SE. Alcohol-related sexual assault victimization among adolescents: prevalence, characteristics, and correlates. *J Stud Alcohol Drugs.* 2008;69:39–48.

52. Brecklin LR, Forde DR. A meta-analysis of rape education programs. *Violence Vict.* 2001;16:303–321.

53. Take Back the Night Web site. http://www.takebackthenight.org/. Accessed November 22, 2009.

54. A Long Walk Home Web site. http://www.alongwalkhome.org/programs.htm. Accessed November 22, 2009.

55. Voices of Men Web site. http://www.voicesofmen.org/. Accessed November 22, 2009.

56. Prevention Connection Web site. http://www.preventconnect.org/display/displayHome.cfm. Accessed November 22, 2009.

57. Fogg P. Rape-prevention programs proliferate, but "It's hard to know" whether they work. Chronicle of Higher Education Web site. http://chronicle.com/article/Rape-Prevention-Programs-Pr/49151/. Accessed November 22, 2009.

Chapter 13

Elder Abuse

Charles P. Mouton, MD, MS
Pamela L. Carter-Nolan, PhD, MPH

INTRODUCTION

Elder abuse and mistreatment has been increasingly identified as a significant problem for older adults. With the growing population of older adults and the increasing numbers who live into the oldest ages, elder abuse and mistreatment unfortunately will continue to be a problem that healthcare providers will need to recognize and manage. In this chapter, we focus on the definition, epidemiology, risks, and health outcomes for this category of abuse and suggest some strategies for managing cases of elder abuse and mistreatment.

DEFINITION

Over time, the definition of what we call elder abuse and mistreatment has steadily evolved. The definition incorporates aspects of violence, intentional psychological harm, and intentional neglect. The National Research Council defines abuse as "intentional actions that cause harm or create a serious risk of harm (whether or not harm is intended) to a vulnerable elder by a caregiver or other person who stands in a trust relationship to the elder" or "failure by a caregiver to satisfy the elder's basic needs or to protect the elder from harm."[1] The American Medical Association defines elder abuse as "acts of omission or commission that result in harm or threatened harm to the health or welfare of an older adult."[2] Both of these definitions speak to harm as a key element in the definition. Separate categories of abuse are delineated within this definition. Physical abuse is the infliction of physical pain, injury, or physical coercion, involving at least one act of violence. Verbal abuse is the infliction of mental anguish through yelling, screaming, threatening, humiliating, infantilizing, or provoking intentional fear.[1,2]

In addition to actual violence against older adults, lack of caring for a dependent older adult has been classified as elder neglect. A proposed definition of elder neglect is the failure to provide services necessary to maintain physical and mental health, namely (1) failure to protect from abuse/exploitation, (2) failure to exercise care (reasonable caregiver), and (3) failure to provide adequate medical or personal care.[1] This definition assumes that the elder victim is dependent on a caregiver to provide the necessary service. However, self-neglect deserves special consideration. Some experts view self-neglect as a separate construct apart from elder abuse and mistreatment. Others view self-neglect as a special category of elder neglect. For this chapter, we do not discuss self-neglect as a category of elder abuse and mistreatment.

EPIDEMIOLOGY

Between 820,000 and 1.9 million older individuals experience maltreatment annually.[3,4] Women are identified as victims in two-thirds of reported elder abuse cases. Only in abandonment cases do men clearly predominate. In a community-based sample of older adults, Pillemer[5] reported that the prevalence of abuse in older adults was 3.2%. More recently, the National Elder Abuse Incidence Study (NEAIS) found that approximately 450,000 older adults were abused and/or neglected during 1996.[3] In this study, women were victims in 76.3% of reports of emotional/psychological abuse, 71.4% of physical abuse, 63.0% of financial/material exploitation, and 60.0% of neglect. Both studies detected abuse in functionally dependent older adults receiving care. Few studies have focused on abuse in functionally independent adults. Mouton et al[6] showed that 11.1% of functionally independent older women were abused in the past year, with a 5% 3-year incidence. Fisher and Regan[7] reported even higher rates, with 47% of women older than 60 years reporting abuse since age 55. However, it is unclear if late-life abuse has the same mental health effects as abuse in younger victims.

Violence is a stressful event that has a negative effect on an elder's psychological well-being. In younger age groups, victims of intimate partner violence (IPV) are at increased risk for psychological problems.[6] Older female victims are twice as more likely to have a psychiatric diagnosis and 1.7–4.6 times more likely to develop an anxiety disorder, a mood disorder, or an eating disorder.[7] Female victims are more than three times as likely to report poor overall mental health and lower vitality.[6,8] Abused women are 2.4–3 times more likely to report depression.[7,9–12] In addition to the direct effects, abuse may negatively impact the factors that improve psychological well-being (i.e., isolation from other social supports).[13]

Coping with the stress of violence may be a key factor mitigating the mental health effects of violence in older adults. Resilience of older adults mitigates the negative impact of stressors such as abuse.[14,15] This optimistic view is one of the key elements in resilience following a traumatic life event and is important for psychological well-being.[16-19] Additionally, poor coping skills and lack of optimism toward the future are correlated with depression ($r = -0.42$) and alcohol use ($r = -0.11$).[18]

High levels of social support also have a favorable effect on psychological outcomes from abuse.[20] High levels of abuse are correlated with a lack of social support in battered women. Moreover, the adverse mental health effects of abuse are mitigated by high social support (relative risk [RR]: 0.5 vs low social support).[20]

Theories

Several theories have been proposed to explain why elder abuse and mistreatment occur. They typically relate to socioenvironmental factors, victim factors, and relationships with an elder's caregiver. Regarding the elderly victims of abuse, theories such as social isolation suggest that an elder who becomes isolated from his/her community is at risk for mistreatment due to lack of a social network.[1] This social isolation is thought to provide the "breeding ground" that allows all family violence (FV) to remain hidden. Because detection by informal associations with friends or relatives can uncover abuse, it is hypothesized that families with strong social networks are less likely to perpetrate elder abuse.[20] Certain personal characteristics relate to the potential victimization of an older adult. Having cognitive impairment and dementia, mental illness, alcohol and/or substance abuse, poor physical function, being female and nonwhite have been reported to promote victimization.[1] Another individual level factor that may contribute to victimization is the relationship between the exposure to violence in childhood and subsequent elder abuse, although this is not yet well understood.

Caregiver Stress

Once thought to be a major cause and predictor of elder abuse and mistreatment, the caregiver stress theory of elder mistreatment suggests that when a caregiver is overwhelmed by the needs of a frail elder, the caregiver may have an aggressive, often violent, response to the elder's needs.[21] The caregiver also may be so overwhelmed that she or he withdraws from providing for the needs of the frail elder. However, case comparison studies have failed to show higher rates of greater caregiver stress in abusive situations.[21] These studies suggest that many caregivers have adequate coping mechanisms for the stress of caregiving, whereas others do not cope as well. Thus, it is not necessarily the stress of caregiving but the caregiver's abilities to cope that underlie the violent behavior.

HEALTH EFFECTS

From a healthcare standpoint, elder abuse and mistreatment are often unrecognized causes of morbidity. In older women, violence results in poorer physical and mental health.[22] Regarding specific illness, elder abuse has been associated with depressive disorders and symptoms, functional decline and frailty, cognitive decline, and a variety of acute injuries ranging from fractures to pressure ulcers.[23,24] Although less well studied in older victims, stress-related conditions, such as elevated blood pressure, anxiety, gastrointestinal syndromes, and genitourinary problems, have been reported to be associated with elder abuse and mistreatment.[24]

RISK FACTORS

Several factors have been cited as predisposing risks for elder abuse. Elders with dementia or cognitive impairment who exhibit disruptive behavior are at increased risk of physical abuse. Elders who suffer from depression, other serious mental health issues, or physical incapacity are more like to suffer from neglect. Elders who have poor mental and physical health and social isolation are more likely to become a victim of financial abuse. Perpetrators of elder abuse are more likely to suffer from mental illness or substance abuse disorders or are dependent (usually financially) on the victim. Any history of violence in the past within the family can increase the risk of abuse.[3,5]

SIGNS AND SYMPTOM OF ELDER MISTREATMENT

In general, the appearance of an older adult can provide clues to the possibility of elder abuse and neglect. If the elder's clothing is inappropriate, soiled, or in disrepair, if there is poor hygiene or signs of wasting, or if there are signs of compromised nutrition and skin integrity, elder abuse or elder mistreatment (EM) should be suspected. Specific signs and symptoms may be linked to particular categories of elder abuse.

Physical Abuse

Physical abuse has both classical and subtle signs in the elderly. Classical signs, including bruises or welts in various healing stages, especially bilaterally or on the inner arms or thighs, fractures, especially in various healing stages, cigarette, rope, chain, or chemical burns, lacerations and abrasions on face, lips, or eyes, bruising, bleeding, hemorrhages beneath the scalp as a consequence of hair pulling, or trauma around the genitalia or rectum are obvious signs of injury related to physical abuse. However, more subtle signs such as anxiety or nervousness in the presence of caregiver, excessive deference to the caregiver, repeated, unexplained, or inconsistently explained falls or injuries requiring emergency department visits, head injuries, hair loss, unusual discharges, delays in seeking treatment, inconsistent follow-up, or constant switching among doctors may be signs of physical abuse. Additionally, any statements about abuse by the patient must be considered an indication of abuse until proven otherwise.[25,26]

The emergency department, home visits, and the private office are important settings for EM assessment. Every effort should be made to not simply treat and release patients whose situation merits further assessment and intervention. Safety concerns should be paramount in the assessment. Astute emergency personnel can identify cases in which there may be serious safety problems in the caregiving situation.

Sexual abuse is a particular type of physical abuse of the elderly. A relatively understudied phenomenon, most reported cases of sexual abuse of the elderly occur within a professional caregiver relationship, such as long-term care.[27] Men usual predominate as perpetrators (often when they are the caregivers), and, if rape occurs, the health provider should approach the patient as she or he would any other rape victim.

Psychological Abuse

Signs of psychological or emotional abuse may often be difficult to detect in a patient encounter. Caregivers often accompany the patient to office visits. When a caregiver demonstrates impatience, irritability, or makes demeaning statements toward the patient, these should be considered as reason for concern about the occurrence of psychological abuse. However, frequently only subtle signs are present in cases of psychological abuse. Signs such as ambivalence of patient to caregiver, high levels of anxiety, fearfulness, or anger, unexpected depression, or withdrawal may all indicate psychological abuse. When an older adult, particularly one who is dependent on someone else, demonstrates lack of adherence to a treatment regimen or has frequently canceled appointments, this should raise the suspicion of possible elder mistreatment. Frequent requests for sedating medication for either the elderly patient or the caregiver also may be a sign of potential abuse.[28]

Neglect

Older adults who have significant cognitive and/or physical impairment require caregiver support for their daily activities. This requirement for caregiver support puts the dependent elder at risk for neglect. Signs of caregiver neglect include the presence of joint contractures, cellulitis, decubitus ulcers, rashes, dehydration or malnutrition, diarrhea, fecal impaction, urine burns, or depression. As with other forms of abuse, signs of neglect may be subtle, such as failure to seek treatment in response to an obvious disease, use of medication that is inadequate, excessive, or otherwise inappropriate, repeated falls, or repeated hospital admissions. Some advocates have considered any pressure ulcer to be a sign of neglect; however, some pressure ulcers may be unavoidable. Again, if the patient makes statements about neglect, the clinician should take these seriously.

Financial Exploitation

A relatively recently recognized problem, financial abuse of older adults, has been drawing increasing attention. Signs suggestive of this form of abuse include the inability of older adults with financial means to be able to afford medication, the inability of the older patient to account for money and property or to pay for essential care, and/or a recent marked disparity between the patient's living conditions or appearance and his or her assets.[1] Often victims of financial abuse report that caregivers and family demand money or goods in exchange for caregiving or other services. Older adults are targets for financial scams that lead to loss of money or property. Abuse should be suspected if there is an unexplained loss of Social Security/pension checks. If an older adult make statements about exploitation, it should be taken as a sign of possible financial abuse.

Abandonment

Although often thought of as a subset of neglect, abandonment is a sign of elder abuse and neglect. Abandonment occurs when the dependent older patient is left alone without adequate arrangements for care. It is manifested by sudden withdrawal of care or sudden departure of the caregiver. Obviously, when older victims are isolated, the impact can be life threatening. The risks of abandonment are similar to those of neglect except abandonment victims are more likely to be male than female.

SELF-NEGLECT

Originally discussed as a form of elder abuse and mistreatment, self-neglect has come under increasing scrutiny as a separate problem from elder abuse.

The evaluation by health providers focuses on other patient attributes. Signs of self-neglect are the same as neglect, but there is no caregiver responsible for the elder. Health professionals have an additional role in self-neglect cases to assess the patient's capacity to understand the risks, benefits, and consequences of accepting or enduring mistreatment.[29] Because the current standard is for health professionals to honor the patient's right to autonomy and self-determination, self-neglect becomes a difficult situation to manage. Arguably, if the patient is able to make his or her own decisions, health provider intervention contrary to the patients' choice is generally inappropriate.

ASSESSMENT

The key tools for addressing elder abuse and mistreatment are routine screening and detection. Initial and routine periodic assessment of older adults for abuse exposure is currently the best method for detecting abuse. Although the US Preventive Services Task Force (USPTF) has not recommended for or against this type of screening, health professionals should consider the value of abuse screening in their patient populations.

In screening for elder abuse, the following preliminary questions can be used:

- Has anyone at home (or in your living setting) ever hurt you?
- Are you afraid of anyone in your family (or environment)?
- Has anyone ever scolded or threatened you?
- Are you receiving enough care at home (or wherever you live)?

If an affirmative response is given to any of these questions, a more formal assessment using one of the standardized instruments, such as the Elder Assessment Instrument or the Brief Abuse Screen for the Elderly, should be done (see Chapter 16 on screening for violence).

As with all other victims, care needs to be taken when questioning an older victim about any form of abuse. The victim should be questioned separately and alone, away from a suspected perpetrator. The general questions listed above can begin the conversation. The healthcare provider should avoid provoking suspicion of the suspected perpetrator to preventing possible retaliation.

INTERVENTION

Prevention

Addressing prevention of elder abuse and mistreatment is typically focused on identifying and mitigating risk factors. Avoiding social isolation and providing support to dependent elders are some general approaches to recognize and prevent the occurrence of elder abuse and mistreatment.

Social Support Services

Health providers need to be aware of, and have the ability to activate, social services for their elderly patients. Referral to case management services, home health care, inpatient and home respite services, and homemaker services are just a few of the support services that can help a dependent elder avoid problems of neglect or self-neglect. Many disease-specific support groups, such as the Alzheimer's Association, are available to provide support and education to caregivers.

MANAGEMENT

The initial focus in the management of abuse is to ensure the safety of the older victim. Removing the older adult from the abusive environment often is necessary. If the older adult is returning to that environment, a safety plan should be developed, discussed with the patient and safe family members, friends, or elder advocates, and put into place.

The time of abuse disclosure also represents an opportunity to educate the older victim about abuse and mistreatment management. Helping older adults understand that these behaviors are abusive, reassuring them that they do not deserve to be treated this way, and educating them about the likelihood of escalation in the future are helpful in managing the impact of abuse on them. Occasionally, violence may be part of a lifelong pattern of interaction between an elder and his or her caregiver. It is similar to "common couple violence" in Johnson's typology of intimate partner violence (IPV).[30] These situations may be amenable to counseling and conflict resolution strategies.

When health providers suspect an older individual is a victim of abuse, they should consider reporting the abuse to an official state agency. Mandatory reporting laws that require the reporting of suspected cases of elder abuse exist in 45 states (including the District of Columbia). Five states do not require mandatory reporting, but each has a mechanism to report and investigate cases of suspected elder abuse if reported. For older adults who are unable to communicate, clinicians should remain vigilant for the signs of abuse mentioned previously. Clear, precise descriptions of any injuries or suspicious behaviors should be documented objectively. The record of the clinical observations may be an essential part of an investigation concerning whether abuse or mistreatment has occurred.

SUMMARY

Elder abuse and mistreatment continues to be an important problem in the care of older adults. Healthcare providers should be vigilant to detect the signs and symptoms of abuse. Selected screening instruments can be applied to identify elderly victims of abuse and mistreatment. Use of these instruments can help providers intervene early to reduce the impact of exposure to elder abuse and mistreatment.

REFERENCES

1. Bonnie RJ, Wallace RB, eds. *Elder Mistreatment: Abuse, Neglect, and Exploitation in an Aging America.* National Research Council, Committee on National Statistics and Committee on Law and Justice, Division of Behavioral and Social Sciences and Education. Washington, DC: The National Academies Press; 2003.
2. American Medical Association diagnostic and treatment guidelines on domestic violence. *Arch Fam Med.* 1992;1(1):39–47.
3. The National Center on Elder Abuse. *The National Elder Abuse Incidence Study.* Final Report. Washington, DC: Administration for Children and Families and the Administration on Aging, DHHS; 1998.
4. Tatara T, Toshio T, Kuzmeskus L. *Summaries of Statistical Data on Elder Abuse in Domestic Settings for FY 95 and FY 96.* Washington, DC: National Center on Elder Abuse; 1997.
5. Pillemer K, Finkelhor D. The prevalence of elder abuse: a random sample survey. *Gerontologist.* 1988;28:51–57.
6. Mouton CP, Rodabough RJ, Rovi SL, et al. Prevalence and 3-year incidence of abuse among postmenopausal women. *Am J Public Health.* 2004;94:605–612.
7. Fisher BS, Regan SL. The extent and frequency of abuse in the lives of older women and their relationship with health outcomes. *Gerontologist.* 2006;46(2):200–209.
8. Lown E, Vega W. Intimate partner violence and health: self-assessed health, chronic health, and somatic symptoms among Mexican American women. *Psychosom Med.* 2001;63:352–360.
9. Danielson K, Moffit T, Caspi A, Silva P. Comorbidity between abuse of an adult and DSM-III-R mental disorders: evidence from an epidemiology study. *Am J Psychiatry.* 1998;155:131–133.
10. Wagner P, Mongan P. Validating the concept of abuse. *Arch Fam Med.* 1998;7:25–32.
11. Petersen R, Gazmaranian J, Clark K. Partner violence: implication for health and community setting. *Womens Health Issues.* 2001;11:116–125.
12. Leserman J, Li Z, Drossman A, Hu Y. Selected symptoms associated with sexual and physical abuse history among female patients with gastrointestinal disorders: the impact on subsequent health care visits. *Psychol Med.* 1998;28:417–425.
13. Roberts G, Williams G, Lawrence J, Raphael B. How domestic violence affects women's mental health. *Women Health.* 1998;28:117–129.
14. Jaffe P, Wolfe D, Wilson S, Zak L. Emotional and physical health problems of battered women. *Can J Psychiatry.* 1986;31:625–654.
15. Coker A, Smith P, Thompson M, McKeown R, Davis K. Social support protects against the negative effects of partner violence on mental health. *J Womens Health Gend Based Med.* 2002;11:465–476.

16. Baltes PB, Baltes MM. Psychological perspectives on successful aging: the model of selective optimization with compensation. In: Baltes PB, Baltes MM, eds. *Successful Aging: Perspectives from the Behavioral Sciences.* Cambridge, MA: Cambridge University Press;1990.

17. Ryff CD, Singer B, Love GD, Essex MJ. Resilience in adulthood and later life: defining features and dynamic process. In: Lomranz J, ed. *Handbook of Aging and Mental Health: An Integrative Approach.* New York, NY: Plenum Press, 1998:69–96.

18. Taylor JY. Moving from surviving to thriving: African American women recovering from intimate male partner abuse. *Res Theory Nurs Pract.* 2004;18(1):35–50.

19. Bowen DJ, Morisca AA, Meischke H. Measures and correlates of resilience. *Women Health.* 2003;38(2):65–76.

20. Scheier M, Carver C, Bridges M. Distinguishing optimism from neuroticism (and trait anxiety, self-mastery and self-esteem): a reevaluation of the life orientation test. *J Pers Soc Psychol.* 1994;67:1063–1078.

21. Sears SF, Serber ER, Lewis TS, et al. Do positive health expectations and optimism relate to quality-of-life outcomes for the patient with an implantable cardioverter defibrillator? *J Cardiopulm Rehabil.* 2004;24(5):324–331.

22. Comijs HC, Jonker C, van Tilburg W, Smit JH. Hostility and coping capacity as risk factors of elder mistreatment. *Soc Psychiatry Psychiatr Epidemiol.* 1999;34:48–52.

23. Phillips L, Torres de Ardon E, Briones G. Abuse of female caregivers by care recipients: another form of elder abuse. *J Elder Abuse Negl.* 2000;12(3/4):123–144.

24. Mouton C. Intimate partner violence and health status among older women. *Violence Against Women.* 2003;9(12):1465–1477.

25. Lachs MS. Screening for family violence: what's an evidence-based doctor to do? *Ann Intern Med.* 2004;140:399–400.

26. Lachs MS, Williams C, O'Brien S, Horwitz R. Risk factors for reported elder abuse and neglect: a nine-year observational cohort study. *Gerontologist.* 1997;37(4):469–474.

27. Teaster P, Roberto K. Sexual abuse of older adults: APS cases and outcomes. *Gerontologist.* 2004;44(6):788–796.

28. Levine J. Elder neglect and abuse: a primer for primary care physicians. *Geriatrics.* 2003;58(10):37–44.

29. Perel-Levin S. *Discussing Screening for Elder Abuse at Primary Health Care Level.* Geneva, Switzerland: World Health Organization; 2008.

30. Johnson MP. *A Typology of Domestic Violence: Intimate Terrorism, Violent Resistance, and Situational Couple Violence.* Lebanon, NH: Northwestern University Press, University Press of New England; 2008.

Chapter 14

Psychological Problems Associated with Family Violence

Anantha Shekhar, MD, PhD

INTRODUCTION

Intimate partner violence (IPV), also known as domestic violence (DV) and family violence (FV), has incidences that range from 6% to 23%, with a lifetime prevalence from 21% to 55% in various populations, and it can result in a wide range of emotional problems. Post-traumatic stress disorder (PTSD), major depressive disorder (MDD), panic attacks, and generalized anxiety disorder (GAD) are commonly seen in people experiencing IPV. These syndromes are all twice as common in women as in men. Differential diagnosis includes other anxiety disorders, dissociative disorder, or seizures due to traumatic brain injury. Treatment approaches include serotonergic antidepressants, anticonvulsants, and psychotherapy. Complications and comorbid conditions include substance abuse, cognitive difficulties, and a worsened prognosis for many concomitant medical conditions. Early diagnosis and intervention are key to preventing chronic disorders and comorbidities.

Interpersonal trauma, even when it occurs sporadically as in accidents or assaults, can have devastating and lifelong adverse effects. When such traumas occur in intimate personal circumstances and often repeatedly, as is frequently seen in IPV, the psychiatric sequelae tend to be quite chronic and severe. IPV can be inflicted on a person in a variety of ways, including physical, sexual, emotional, or financial abuse. It is a major public health problem and can have long-term health consequences for "direct victims" who experience it; however, it also can have severe consequences for "passive victims," such as children who witness it. The incidence of this problem varies depending on the populations being studied. Recent data obtained from women attending general medical practices revealed that the prevalence of physical or sexual IPV in the past year from a partner or ex-partner ranged from 6% to 23%, and lifetime prevalence varied from 21% to 55%.[1]

PATHOPHYSIOLOGY

From a bioevolutionary perspective, we have developed anxiety reactions as an alarm system that occurs in response to danger or threat. Victims of IPV, confronted with the threat of interpersonal violence, develop a variety of defensive responses to counter these dangers, which may include escape behaviors, avoidance, aggressive defense, submission, or a combination of behaviors. For each type of defensive behavior, there is a corresponding physiological substrate to support the activation and mobilization of resources. The sympathetic activity that is characterized as the fight-or-flight mode is neither dangerous nor harmful but is intended to be aversive, so that a response will be initiated, resulting in a defensive maneuver.

Anxiety, when viewed as an alarm system, has three necessary components: the ability to detect a threat, the ability to identify the threat as a danger, and the ability to respond appropriately to the danger. Under normal circumstances, such a system will be set for a sensitivity that is balanced between the costs of false alarms, such as mounting an escape response when there is no danger, versus the cost of missing a true alarm and failing to respond to an actual danger. Given the relatively low costs of false versus true alarms in the context of danger, a biologic alarm system will, therefore, be biased towards high sensitivity (i.e., "better safe than sorry"). In addition, the strength of the response will be directly related to the strength of the perceived threat. However, with repeated expectation of danger, the system may maintain a constant level of "hypervigilance." When even the slightest danger cues are detected as present, the system then intensifies into a "response" status, whereupon the body is mobilized for a direct action expressed as a panic attack or withdrawal.

IPV can induce dysregulation in any of the three components of threat detection, threat interpretation, or threat response. A state of persistent hypervigilance will result in an over-detection of threats; catastrophic thinking patterns can result in false perceptions of threat; and avoidance and escape behaviors may become overused, resulting in maintenance of fears. For example, GAD is a perturbed alarm system, whose threshold for threat detection is set too low. PTSD and acute stress disorder (ASD) develop from the overwhelming activation of the response component of the alarm system, when it continues to be triggered despite the cessation of the true danger. Panic disorder may start as a dysregulation of the response system (i.e., panic attacks following acute trauma), but soon becomes entrenched in problems of catastrophic interpretation of the threat. Following repeated exposure to a feared stimulus (threat detection), threat interpretation can become catastrophically misperceived as overly dangerous and inescapable, resulting in severe depression. This chapter reviews some of the potential psychiatric disorders that may be seen following IPV and discusses some basic issues of diagnosis and management of such disorders. In the following section, each of the psychiatric disorders that can be seen in victims of IPV is reviewed for its essential and defining features.

COMMON PSYCHIATRIC PROBLEMS

Acute Stress/Post-traumatic Stress Disorder

Acute stress and PTSD are the most common sequelae of IPV and occur following the experience of a "true alarm." Difficulties integrating a traumatic experience in one's life generally occur when the traumatic event consists of a perceived or actual threat of death or physical integrity to oneself or someone else. Most persons exposed to these types of events experience transient reactions to the trauma, usually some form of reoccurrence of the trauma (images, thoughts, dreams, flashbacks), symptoms of dissociation (numbing of emotion, reduction in awareness, derealization, depersonalization, amnesia), increased arousal (difficulty sleeping, irritability, exaggerated startle response, motor restlessness, poor concentration), and avoidance of stimuli associated with the trauma. When these symptoms begin to cause significant distress or disruption in the person's life, the traumatic response crosses the threshold into ASD. However, studies have indicated that for most people who experience a single or brief "threat," these traumatic symptoms often begin to resolve within a month. When they persist for longer than 4 weeks, the diagnosis becomes PTSD, indicating a failure of the alarm system to shut off.

The *Diagnostic and Statistical Manual of Psychiatric Disorders*, 4th edition (*DSM-IV*),[2] provides separate definitions for "trauma" and the two psychiatric syndromes arising from a traumatic experience: the more common and short-duration anxiety disorder known as ASD, and PTSD, the longer-lasting, more severe anxiety syndrome. The concept of "trauma" needed to be defined because, although most subjects develop acute or post-traumatic stress disorders following the experience of an actual threat of death or physical integrity, it can also arise from a perceived threat or witnessing harm to someone else, which arouses a severe experience of horror (*DSM-IV*). Subjects who have experienced trauma report transient distressing reactions, usually some form of re-experiencing of the trauma (images, thoughts, dreams, flashbacks); symptoms of dissociation (numbing of emotion, reduction in awareness, derealization, depersonalization, and amnesia); increased arousal (difficulty sleeping, irritability, exaggerated startle response, motor restlessness, poor concentration); and avoidance of stimuli associated with the trauma. If such responses last a few days, but resolve within 4 weeks, a diagnosis of ASD is given. However, if these symptoms last longer than 4 weeks, a diagnosis of PTSD can be made.

Generalized Anxiety Disorder (GAD)

Often characterized as the "basic anxiety disorder," GAD is defined by worry that is pervasive and uncontrollable to the extent that it interferes with daily functioning or causes marked distress. In defining GAD, the main concern is to discriminate pathological worry from the normal adaptive level of worry. Some of the key findings from epidemiological studies of GAD were that pathological worry and normal worry can be differentiated based on the amount of time consumed with worry, the person's ability to "suppress" or distract oneself away from the worry, as well as by accompanying physiological symptoms. Excessive worry was discriminated from normal worry by being associated with at least three of the following symptoms: feeling keyed up/on edge, restlessness, easy fatiguability, difficulty concentrating, irritability, and difficulty sleeping. Again, consistent with a model of hypervigilance or "heightened threat detection," pathological worry also was associated with duration, because "normal worry" typically resolves with the cessation of an episode of stress while pathological worry persists despite stress resolution. The diagnostic criteria for GAD were therefore extended to a requirement of 6 months' duration.

Panic Disorder

The *DSM-IV* provides separate definitions for panic attacks and panic disorder. This is significant because most individuals who meet criteria for other anxiety disorders, such as PTSD, also present with secondary panic attacks.[2] The panic attack criteria require a sudden episode of distress, with at least 4 of 13 key panic symptoms, and the "episode" itself must peak within 10 minutes. The 13 key symptoms of a panic attack, primarily due to autonomic overactivity, are: heart palpitations/pounding, sweating, trembling/shaking, shortness of breath, feeling of choking, chest pain/discomfort, nausea/abdominal distress, dizziness/unsteadiness, derealization, fear of losing control/going crazy, fear of dying, paresthesias, and chills/hot flushes. With this separate definition, panic attacks are viewed as symptoms that can occur in the context of a perceived imminent, severe threat; thus, they may be diagnosed as occurring within any anxiety disorder, or, if occurring in isolation, may be a normal response to acute stress in 20% of adults.

DIAGNOSIS AND DIFFERENTIAL DIAGNOSIS

The most important challenges are the timely recognition of IPV cases and the ability to address barriers to asking victims about IPV and to encourage appropriate responses to disclosure and referral to specialists. Practitioners should routinely integrate questions about abuse into medical evaluations. Other components of the intervention should include a seamless referral pathway to an IPV advocate. However, once a potential psychiatric sequela is suspected, the following diagnostic evaluation should be considered to clarify possible psychiatric diagnoses.

DSM-IV diagnosis of PTSD is usually made by eliciting the typical features in a clinical interview: the occurrence of traumatic experience followed by symptoms of re-experiencing, hyperarousal, emotional numbing, and avoidance.[2] If the symptoms have lasted less than 4 weeks, a diagnosis of ASD can be made. The diagnosis of PTSD requires persistence of symptoms for at least 4 weeks. If seen in an emergency department during or immediately following an acute traumatic event, it is important to inquire about acute dissociation or numbing, because these may predict a greater likelihood of developing PTSD. Such subjects should be referred to appropriate follow-up facilities to treat any emerging symptoms of ASD and, if possible, to prevent the development of PTSD.

The differential diagnoses for PTSD are usually suggested by atypical features in either the history or physical examination. Beyond basic chemistries, a neurologic workup with electroencephalograph (EEG) and magnetic resonance imaging (MRI) may be indicated if the history is suggestive of head trauma or seizures. More extensive evaluations with sleep studies or neuroendocrine tests may be indicated in some patients.

Diagnosis of panic attacks and panic disorder also are made by clinical interview. If seen in an emergency department during or immediately following an acute panic attack, it is important to elicit information about sudden onset, rapid peaking, and multisystem symptoms (cardiac, respiratory, neurologic, gastrointestinal, and psychological) of the attack in the absence of other serious medical conditions. Common signs observed on physical examination of a subject during an acute panic attack, most often in the emergency department, include sinus tachycardia, hyperventilation, and mild systolic hypertension. Patients seen in outpatient settings with a typical history suggestive of panic disorder may show mild resting tachycardia or tachypnea.

Differential diagnoses for panic disorder are usually suggested by a good history and physical examination. Typically, the patient is a healthy young individual with very few cardiovascular risk factors. Therefore, any further work-up beyond basic chemistries, electrocardiogram, and urine toxicology should only be performed if compelling risk factors are elicited in the history or physical. Similarly, beyond baseline thyroid functions in women, an extensive endocrine work-up should only be undertaken if indicated by physical signs.

TREATMENT AND CLINICAL CARE

Subjects with psychiatric disorders emerging from IPV can be relatively difficult to engage in treatment, with fewer than 50% of them entering therapy. Various psychosocial barriers to treatment have been noted. The first and the most important step in successfully treating such subjects is the development of a trusting relationship with the health professional. Cognitive behavior therapy (CBT), especially when instituted soon after trauma, may be a very effective treatment.[3,4] Other types of psychological treatments such as eye movement desensitization and reprocessing also have shown promise.[4] In addition to traditional CBT techniques to manage psychiatric symptoms, therapy for these patients needs to be augmented with additional interventions, such as ensuring safety and teaching skills to access important community resources and to establish support systems for themselves and their dependents.[5]

Currently the selective serotonin reuptake inhibitors (SSRIs), such as paroxetine (Paxil®) and sertraline (Zoloft®), are approved by the US Food and Drug Administration (FDA) and are considered first-line medication treatments for PTSD, GAD, panic, and MDD.[6,7] Thus, SSRIs can be used as the ideal treatment for many subjects who often have comorbid conditions, such as PTSD, depression, panic, and GAD.[7] Unfortunately, a substantial number of patients only respond partially to SSRIs, and others may develop intolerable side effects during the initiation of these medications. There is evidence that adding α-adrenergic receptor antagonists, such as prazosin, may be helpful in treating symptoms of hyperarousal and sleep disturbances. Another effective drug group, which is used less often now but could be second-line drugs, is the tricyclic antidepressants (TCAs). The TCAs cause greater weight gain and anticholinergic side effects, but, of greater concern, is their lethal toxicity in overdose.

Some anticonvulsant drugs, such valproate (Depakote®) and gabapentin (Neurontin®), also are employed to treat some symptoms of PTSD. Benzodiazepines and hypnotics are still widely used adjuncts for short periods of symptomatic relief, but they need to be closely monitored for potential dependence. In particularly resistant cases, some studies have reported benefits from the use of atypical antipsychotic drugs, such as olanzapine (Zyprexa®), as adjuncts to standard treatments. More recently, novel pharmacologic agents that enhance conditioning, such as D-cycloserine, have been used in conjunction with psychological treatments.[8]

The use of benzodiazepines in the treatment of anxiety disorders is worth some additional comments. Short-term benzodiazepines are widely used in treating these patients, and the "high-potency" benzodiazepines, like lorazepam, alprazolam, and clonazepam, are preferred now in clinical practices. These benzodiazepines have the benefits of a favorable side-effect profile and a rapid onset of action, showing improvement within a week in one study. Drawbacks to benzodiazepines, however, include the development of physiologic dependence with sustained use and the risk of abuse in persons predisposed to substance abuse. In contrast, SSRIs have a very low abuse or dependence potential. Recent work has shown that coadministration of a benzodiazepine, such as clonazepam or alprazolam, with SSRIs, such as sertraline, accelerates the response of patients with moderate to severe panic disorder and may reduce early antidepressant-related stimulation. Thus, benzodiazepines may be effectively used for short-term stabilization and SSRIs for longer-term management/control of symptoms.[9]

In summary, severe, chronic psychiatric disorders can develop following the experience of IPV. It is important to recognize the potential for these long-term complications while evaluating patients in emergency departments or in the office setting after a recent experience of such violence and to have a comprehensive approach to manage these patients.[10]

REFERENCES

1. Gregory A, Ramsay J, Agnew-Davies R, et al. Primary care identification and referral to improve safety (IRIS) of women experiencing domestic violence: protocol for a pragmatic cluster randomised controlled trial. *BMC Public Health.* 2010;10:54.

2. American Psychiatric Association. *Diagnostic and Statistical Manual of Psychiatric Disorders.* 4th ed. Washington, DC: American Psychiatric Association; 1994.

3. Sijbrandij M, Olff M, Reitsma JB, Carlier IV, de Vries MH, Gersons BP. Treatment of acute post-traumatic stress disorder with brief cognitive behavioral therapy: a randomized controlled trial. *Am J Psychiatry.* 2007;164(1):82–90.

4. Ponniah K, Hollon SD. Empirically supported psychological treatments for adult acute stress disorder and posttraumatic stress disorder: a review. *Depress Anxiety.* 2009;26(12):1086–1109.

5. Johnson DM, Zlotnick C. HOPE for battered women with PTSD in domestic violence shelters. *Prof Psychol Res Pr.* 2009;40(3):234–241.

6. Stein DJ, Ipser JC, Seedat S. Pharmacotherapy for post-traumatic stress disorder (PTSD). *Cochrane Database Syst Rev.* 2006;(1):CD002795.

7. Dell'Osso B, Buoli M, Baldwin DS, Altamura AC. Serotonin norepinephrine reuptake inhibitors (SNRIs) in anxiety disorders: a comprehensive review of their clinical efficacy. *Hum Psychopharmacol.* 2010;25(1):17–29.

8. Cukor J, Spitalnick J, Difede J, Rizzo A, Rothbaum BO. Emerging treatments for PTSD. *Clin Psychol Rev.* 2009;29(8):715–726.

9. Goddard AW, Brouette T, Almai A, Jetty P, Woods SW, Charney D. Early coadministration of clonazepam with sertraline for panic disorder. *Arch Gen Psychiatry.* 2001;58(7):681–686.

10. Olive P. Care for emergency department patients who have experienced domestic violence: a review of the evidence base. *J Clin Nurs.* 2007;16(9):1736–1748.

Chapter 15

Substances of Abuse and Family Violence

Sandra Kamnetz, MD
Mary Beth Plane, MSSW, PhD
Valerie J. Gilchrist, MD

INTRODUCTION

Intimate partner violence (IPV) and other forms of family violence (FV) often coexist with use of alcohol and other substances of abuse. Violence in all forms in the United States is greater among intimate partners when alcohol or drugs of abuse are frequently consumed. In this chapter, violence is broadly defined as the use of intentional emotional, psychological, sexual, or physical force by one partner against another (see Chapter 1). This also includes financial abuse, withholding care and medicine, and child abuse or elder neglect. Spouses, parents, stepparents, children, siblings, elderly relatives, and intimate partners may all be targets of such interpersonal violence.[1] Substance abuse adds a layer of complexity to an already abusive family situation. However, alcohol or drugs used by any partner do *not* cause the violence; they may exacerbate violence that is already happening in the family setting.

ALCOHOL ABUSE AND DEPENDENCE

Over half of the US population drinks alcohol during the course of a month; 5% drink heavily, and 15% report at least one episode of binge-drinking each month. Heavy drinking is defined as two or more drinks per day for men and one drink per day on average for women. Binge-drinking is defined as five or more drinks on a single occasion for men and four or more for women.

Both alcohol dependence and abuse are more prevalent among men, whites, Native Americans, and younger and unmarried adults.[2] Men are twice as likely as women to binge-drink. The prevalence of alcohol use disorders has been found to be higher in primary care settings than in the general population.

Both heavy drinking and binge-drinking are considered alcohol abuse. The definition of alcohol dependence generally relies on the *Diagnostic and Statistical Manual of Mental Disorders*, 4th ed. (*DSM-IV*) of the American Psychiatric Association (APA) and includes such issues as increased tolerance, withdrawal symptoms, impaired control, neglect of social or occupational activities, time spent drinking, and continued use despite alcohol-related consequences.[3] According to a recent review by the Centers for Disease Control and Prevention (CDC),[4] alcohol use and dependence is related to unintentional injuries and two out of three incidents of IPV.[5]

DRUG USE AND ABUSE

Illicit drugs include marijuana/hashish, cocaine and crack, heroin, hallucinogens, inhalants, or illegally obtained or used prescription medications.[6] In 2008, an estimated 20.1 million Americans 12 years or older (8% of the population) used an illicit drug during the past month. This figure has remained stable since 2002.[1] Marijuana was the drug of choice for three of four (6.1% of the population) of those using illicit drugs; 3.4% used other substances of abuse, including prescription medications (2.5%). Methamphetamines, cocaine, or hallucinogens were each used by less than 1%.[1]

Rates of past-month illicit drug use varied by age from 3.3% for those 12 or 13 years to the highest rate of 21.5 % among persons 18 to 20 years, decreasing to 1% for those 65 years or older. Current illicit drug use has remained relatively stable across all age groups since 2002.[6]

Screening for Substance Abuse

Although the four-question CAGE[7] (**C**ut back, **A**nnoyance by critics, **G**uilt about drinking, and **E**ye-opening morning drinking) is a good alcohol screening instrument, the following two items conjointly screen for alcohol and other drug problems and have been found to have 80% sensitivity and specificity for detecting current substance use disorders in young and middle-aged adults.[8]

- In the last 12 months, did you ever find yourself drinking or using drugs more than you meant to?
- In the last 12 months, did you ever think that maybe you should cut down on your drinking or drug use?

The following is a single-item alcohol screening tool with 86% sensitivity and specificity for detecting hazardous drinking and alcohol use disorders: "When was the last time you had more than 'X' drinks in one day?" where "X" equals four for women and five for men.[9]

The following is a single-item tool ("In the last 12 months, did you smoke pot, use another street drug, or use a prescription pain-killer, stimulant, or sedative for a non-medical reason?"[10]) that is being used successfully (i.e., identifying abuse correctly) in a large Screening Brief Intervention Referral and Treatment (SBIRT) intervention in the Midwest.[10] Sensitivity and specificity have not yet been established.

INTIMATE PARTNER VIOLENCE

Relationship Between Substance Use and Intimate Partner Violence

Significant features common to both IPV and substance abuse include continuation of the behavior despite adverse consequences, preoccupation or obsession with the behavior, and development of tolerance to the behavior. There is a relationship between alcohol intoxication and violence. Individuals with drinking-related social consequences or alcohol dependence symptoms have higher levels of marital discord, fights, and verbal aggression, which could place them at risk for IPV (both as victims and perpetrators). Caetano et al[11] reported that 30–40% of men and 4–24% of women were drinking during violent episodes between couples. A meta-analysis in 2008 by Foran and O'Leary[12] found "a small to moderate effect size between alcohol use/abuse and male-to-female partner violence and a small effect size for the association between alcohol use/abuse and female-to-male partner violence." Although alcohol is a significant cofactor in partner aggression, this does not reduce the responsibility of the perpetrator. Drinking consumption patterns alone are not a predictor of IPV overall; however, alcohol-related problems are.[13] Additionally, one cannot blame the victim for alcohol or drug use because in many cases it may be her only escape from her traumatized life. There are multiple risk factors in any incidence of partner aggression that need to be addressed in any individual case.[12,14] Violent behavior and drug use can result from the same factors (e.g., high sensation seeking) and exist coincidentally. The drugs and violence relationship may coexist when drugs pharmacologically induce violence and/or because violence may be used to obtain drugs.[15]

Women who use drugs are at increased risk of experiencing partner violence.[16] They sometimes describe their use of alcohol and drugs as a mechanism to cope with the abuse, which then can compound their vulnerability to experiencing violence in intimate relationships.[16]

Management of Substance Abuse and IPV

Failure to address IPV issues among substance abusers interferes with treatment effectiveness and contributes to relapse of their substance abuse.[17,18] Issues of safety and isolation need to be addressed for treatment to be successful. Focusing on only the substance abuse without considering the IPV will potentially send a woman back to a high-risk setting, both for more abuse and for relapse. Physical injuries can have long-lasting cognitive, psychological, and physical effects that interfere with the victim's ability to follow a treatment program. Female survivors of male perpetrators may have difficulty accepting treatment or professional services from men. Victimization may cloud patients' attitudes and beliefs about being able to control their lives and their ability to control their alcohol and substance abuse. Victims may have difficulty developing a trusting relationship with providers.[18]

Studies of substance-abusing women in domestic violence shelters found that they generally decreased their use of alcohol and stimulants in the period following their shelter stay. These studies further support the need to help substance-abusing women with finances, housing, and health that are interconnected in complex ways to the violence and substance abuse they are experiencing. Programs for substance abuse treatment, domestic violence, health care, and other agencies need to be coordinated for women to make gains.[16]

CHILD ABUSE

Children living in families in which alcohol and substance abuse occurs are at extremely high risk for being "severely and chronically traumatized."[19] The children of parents who abuse substances are 2.7 times more likely to be abused and 4.2 times more likely to be neglected.[20] Substance abuse by caregivers, including parents, is also associated with more severe physical abuse and as many as two-thirds of all cases of child maltreatment fatalities.[20,21]

Traumatic childhood events (including witnessing parental violence and living with a parent or family member who abuses substances) are correlated not only with childhood risk but also with adult health risk behaviors and diseases.[18,19] Adult respondents who had experienced four or more of these childhood adversities had a 4- to 12-fold increased likelihood of alcoholism, drug abuse, depression, and suicide attempts and a 2- to 4-fold increased likelihood of smoking (including smoking by age 14 years and chronic smoking as adults) and sexually transmitted diseases.[19] They are also more likely to experience future violence.

Children can be affected directly or indirectly by living in a home in which there is active substance abuse. Children who live in a household where there is parental violence or parental substance use can have lifelong psychological sequelae. Substances can be transmitted *in utero*, and affected children may present with prematurity or developmental delays (including fetal alcohol syndrome) that demand resources and parenting expertise that is even more of a challenge to parents who are substance abusers. Battered women may not have the resources to prevent their children's potential exposure to abuse and, furthermore, may resort to use of more drugs or alcohol themselves to help them cope.[19] Pregnancy and childbirth may be an opportune time to intervene in both a violent and substance abuse setting, because women may become concerned about the effect of alcohol or violence on a pregnancy and because many women get routine prenatal care that may offer the opportunity to inquire about risks and offer education and treatment. Children exposed to substances of abuse *in utero* may also be at greater risk of abuse or neglect in the postnatal period.[20]

Children are at risk of being affected by a range of dysfunctional behaviors by substance-abusing parents, including inadequate parenting, mental illness, family violence (FV), and exposure to criminal activities. Substance abuse by parents or other adults in the home puts children at risk for poverty and inadequate financial resources.[20,21] Children may be more likely to be directly physically abused by parents or caregivers who use substances associated with increased aggression, most commonly alcohol and methamphetamine.[12]

In an Australian study of 302 homeless youth, 8% cited familial drug and alcohol use as the critical factor that made them leave home.[22] Children exposed to violence are more likely to experience violence in their adult lives (as either the abuser or the victim); similarly, children exposed to substance abuse are more likely to become substance abusers and start use at an earlier age.[18,20]

Women are often afraid to address alcohol or substance abuse problems for fear of losing custody of their children; however, interventions to reduce problem drinking have been shown to reduce arrests for child abuse.[23] Treatment centers for domestic violence often are equipped to care for children, but treatment facilities for alcohol and substance abuse often are not.[16,18] In general, domestic violence shelters do not have programs to treat alcohol or substance abuse and may not allow substance abusers to reside in the shelters. Alcohol treatment programs usually do not provide services that address IPV. Thus, women attend one program or the other with little cross-referral or related services provided.

ELDER ABUSE

Six percent of older individuals in the general population report abuse.[24] These individuals are at risk for the same forms of violence as are other family members, and alcohol/substance abuse by the perpetrator can worsen their plight. Greenberg et al[25] found 44% of substantiated instances of individuals in which the abusers were identified as having alcohol or drug abuse problems.[25] Several case-control studies in the late 1980s and early 1990s found that abusers of the elderly were disproportionately more likely to have an alcohol use problem, with increased consumption related strongly to physical abuse compared with emotional abuse.[26] Elderly individuals who themselves have in the past or who currently abuse alcohol or drugs may find themselves living with family members who also are substance abusers. The risk for elder abuse also may be increased further because of the challenge of caring for a substance-abusing older person in the setting of the caretaker's own substance abuse.[27] Other risk factors for caregiver abuse include social isolation, mental health diagnoses, alcohol abuse, patient need for a caregiver, patient cognitive impairment, financial dependence of the caregiver on the older adult, and shared living arrangements.[28,29]

As is true for all forms of FV, elder abuse is underreported. A reasonable screen for the risk factor of substance abuse in the family is "Does anyone in your family drink a lot?"[30] If there is substance abuse in the family, clinicians should have a higher index of suspicion for elder abuse, and, if abuse is suspected, they should inquire about family members' substance use. Older adults are more likely to see their primary care physicians than are younger adults and use emergency services twice as often as other age groups, presenting more opportunities for inquiry and detection.[28,31,32]

CLINICAL CONTEXT

Clinicians should use exploratory or screening questions to obtain more information about both potential violence and substance abuse. It is important to inform the patient about the frequency of coexistence of these two conditions. Some examples of questions to use include the following.

Questions

1. Tell me about your alcohol or other substance use.
2. Has it ever been a problem for you . . . or for others in your family?
3. How do differences get resolved in your family?
4. Do you feel safe at home?
5. How do you discipline your children?
6. Do you act differently around your family when you have been drinking or using drugs?
7. Do you ever feel out of control when you are drinking or using drugs?

Refer to Fellow Professionals

Examples include social service agencies, counselors, Alcoholics Anonymous (AA), or other self-help groups. Learn about these resources in your community. Physicians cannot solve these problems alone, and they must do their best to protect the vulnerable. The elderly woman and the children in these scenarios are at risk; as a physician, although legal responsibilities vary by state, you have a responsibility to protect the vulnerable.

Patient Support

Support your patient over time. Leaving an abusive relationship or ending substance abuse is a process that continues, sometimes over a lifetime.

SUMMARY AND CONCLUSIONS

- Substance abuse, especially alcohol abuse, is common.
- Substance abuse increases the risk of all types of FV.
- Concern about either FV or substance abuse should lead to inquiry about the other.
- Treatment of violence and substance abuse needs to be coordinated and concurrent.

REFERENCES

1. Peace at Home. *Domestic Violence: The Facts*. Boston, MA: Peace at Home; 1995.
2. Hasin DS, Stinson FS, Ogburn E, Grant BF. Prevalence, correlates, disability, and comorbidity of DSM-IV alcohol abuse and dependence in the United States. *Arch Gen Psychiatry*. 2007;64(7):830–842.
3. Hasin D. Classification of alcohol use disorders. National Institute on Alcohol Abuse and Alcoholism Web site. http://pubs.niaaa.nih.gov/publications/arh27-1/5-17.htm. Accessed February 13, 2010.

4. Fact sheets. Alcohol use and health. Division of Adult and Community Health, National Center for Chronic Disease Prevention and Health Promotion. Centers for Disease Control and Prevention Web site. http://www.cdc.gov/alcohol/fact-sheets/alcohol-use.htm. Accessed February 13, 2010.

5. Greenfield LA. Alcohol and crime: an analysis of national data on the prevalence of alcohol involvement in crime. Report prepared for the Assistant Attorney General's National Symposium on Alcohol Abuse and Crime. Washington, DC: US Department of Justice; 1998. Office of Justice Programs Web site. http://www.ojp.usdoj.gov/bjs/pub/pdf/ac.pdf. Accessed March 31, 2008.

6. Substance use and dependence following initiation of alcohol or illicit drug Use. National Survey on Drug Use and Health, 2008. Office of Applied Studies Web site. http://www.oas.samhsa.gov/NSDUH/2k8NSDUH/2k8results.cfm#Ch2. Accessed January 10, 2010.

7. Ewing JA. Detecting alcoholism. The CAGE questionnaire. *JAMA.* 1984;252(14):1905-1907.

8. Brown RL, Leonard T, Saunders LA, Papasouliotis O. A two item conjoint screen for alcohol and other drug problems. *J Am Board Fam Pract.* 2001;14(2):95-106.

9. Williams R, Vinson D. Validation of a single screening question for problem drinking. *J Fam Pract.* 2001;50(4)307-312.

10. Brown R. 2010 personal communication.

11. Caetano R, Cunradi C, Clark C, Schafer J. Intimate partner violence and drinking patterns among white, black, and Hispanic couples in the United States. *J Subst Abuse.* 2000;11(2):123-138.

12. Foran H, O'Leary KD. Alcohol and intimate partner violence: a meta-analytic review. *Clin Psychol Rev.* 2008;28(7):1222-1234.

13. Cunradi C, Caetano R, Clark C, Schafer J. Alcohol-related problems and intimate partner violence among white, black, and Hispanic couples in the United States. *Alcohol Clin Exp Res.* 1999;23(9):1492-1501.

14. Murphy CM, Eckhardt CI. *Treating the Abusive Partner: An Individualized Cognitive-Behavioral Approach.* New York, NY: Guilford Press; 2005.

15. Hoaken P, Stewart S. Drugs of abuse and the elicitation of human aggressive behavior. *Addict Behav.* 2003;28:1533-1554.

16. Poole N, Greaves L, Jategaonkar N, McCullough L, Chabot C. Substance use by women using domestic violence shelters. *Subst Use Misuse.* 2008;43(8-9):1129-1150.

17. Fazzone PA, Holton JK, Reed, BG. *Tip 25: Substance Abuse Treatment and Domestic Violence.* Rockville, MD: Substance Abuse and Mental Health Administration; 1997.

18. Miller BA, Wilsnack SC, Cunradi CB. Family violence and victimization: treatment issues for women with alcohol problems. *Alcohol Clin Exp Res.* 2000;24(8):1287-1297.

19. Harris WW, Lieberman AF, Marans S. In the best interests of society. *J Child Psychol Psychiatry.* 2007;48(3):392-411.

20. Wells K. Substance abuse and child maltreatment. *Pediatr Clin North Am.* 2009;56(2):345-362.

21. National Alliance for Drug Endangered Children Web site. http://www.nationaldec.org. Accessed September 13, 2010.

22. Mallett S, Rosenthal D, Keys D. Young people, drug use and family conflict: pathways into homelessness. *J Adolesc.* 2005;28(2):185–199.

23. Dinh-Zarr TB, Goss CW, Heitman E, Roberts IG, DiGuiseppi C. Interventions for preventing injuries in problem drinkers. *Cochrane Database Syst Rev.* 2004;3: CD001857.

24. Cooper C, Selwood A, Livingston G. The prevalence of elder abuse and neglect: a systematic review. *Age Ageing.* 2008;37(2):151–160.

25. Greenberg JR, McKibben M, Raymond JA. Dependent adult children and elder abuse. *J Elder Abuse Negl.* 1990;2:73–86.

26. Bonnie R, Wallace RB, eds. Risk factors for elder mistreatment. In: *Elder Mistreatment: Abuse, Neglect, and Exploitation in an Aging America.* Washington, DC: The National Academies Press; 2003:95.

27. Reis M, Nahmiash D. Validation of the Indicators of Abuse (IOA) Screen. *Gerontologist.* 1998;38(4):471–480.

28. Kleinschmidt KC. Elder abuse: a review. *Ann Emerg Med.* 1997;309(4):463–472.

29. Lachs MS, Pillemer K. Abuse and neglect of elderly persons. *N Engl J Med.* 1995;332(7):437–443.

30. Hwalek MA, Sengstock MC. Assessing the probability of abuse of the elderly: toward the development of a clinical screening instrument. *J Appl Gerontol.* 1986;5:153–173.

31. Spaite DW, Criss EA, Valenzuela TD, Meislin HW, Ross J. Geriatric injury: an analysis of pre-hospital demographics, mechanisms and patterns. *Ann Emerg Med.* 1990;19(12):1418–1421.

32. Carmel S, Anson O, Levin M. Emergency department utilization: a comparative analysis of older-adults, old and old-old patients. *Aging (Milano).* 1990;(2):387–393.

Chapter 16

Screening for Family Violence

Amy S. Gottlieb, MD
Sarina Schrager, MD, MS

INTRODUCTION

A screening program must meet certain criteria to be feasible. The disease that is the focus of the program must have a negative impact on health. In addition, for a screening program to be effective, there should be evidence that an early diagnosis of the condition affects the outcome.[1] A good screening test is defined as one that[1]

- is acceptable to the patient and the practitioner (i.e., is easy to do);
- confers limited risk to the patient at a reasonable cost;
- is accurate (i.e., has a high sensitivity and specificity); and
- can detect the condition at an early stage.

The US Preventive Services Task Force (USPSTF) confers a level I (indeterminate) recommendation for universal screening for family violence (FV) because there is not enough evidence to show that screening, or early detection, alters outcomes.[2] No studies consistently show that early identification of family abuse affects future violent episodes or injuries. Despite this lack of evidence, most professional groups advocate routine screening for FV by healthcare providers because of its high prevalence and significant morbidity and mortality.[3] Violence screening can occur during any clinical encounter, from primary care health maintenance exams to emergency department patient intake evaluations. Routine screening may decrease the stigma of FV by normalizing the discussion of violence. This chapter reviews screening guidelines for the three types of FV: child abuse, intimate partner violence (IPV), and elder abuse.

SCREENING FOR CHILD ABUSE

Screening for child abuse may be challenging. For example, who should be screened, the child or the parent? For young children, asking about abuse or neglect may make them uncomfortable or difficult. If the parent is the abuser, the clinician may not be able to assess for abuse if that person is present during the patient interview. In addition, the abuser may have told the child never to tell anyone about the abuse.

Several instruments are available for child abuse screening in the healthcare setting. However, none has been shown to alter outcomes such as reducing abuse or preventing injuries.[4] Most of the available screening instruments have high sensitivities but low specificities and have not been tested in the general population. No studies have demonstrated any harm from screening.[4] Because it is not reliable to ask young children about abuse, the main screening instruments for child abuse assess whether parents are at risk of abusing their children. Two commonly used screening instruments are the Kempe Family Stress Inventory (KFSI) and the Hawaii Risk Indicators Screening Tool.[5]

The KFSI is a 10-item instrument that evaluates a parent's risk of developing parenting stress.[6] Parenting stress is directly related to the occurrence of child abuse.[4] The KFSI includes questions about the parent's history of personal childhood violence, history of mental illness, substance abuse history, and criminal background. It also includes questions about family stressors and the parent–child relationship (Table 16-1). The KFSI has been

Table 16-1 The Kempe Family Stress Inventory (Child Abuse Screening Tool)

1. Parent is a victim of child abuse or neglect
2. Past history of criminal behavior, mental illness, or substance abuse in parent
3. Previous suspicion of abuse by parent
4. Parent with low self-esteem or social isolation
5. Multiple family stressors or crises
6. Parent with uncontrolled anger
7. Unrealistic expectations of child's behavior
8. Severe punishment of child
9. Child with challenging behaviors or parent's perception of challenging behaviors
10. Unwanted pregnancy or other risk for poor bonding

Source: Adapted from Korfmacher J. The Kempe Family Stress Inventory: a review. *Child Abuse Negl.* 2000;24(1):129–140.

tested in pregnant women to predict future risk of child maltreatment, and it predicted maltreatment at 1 and 2 years after testing (positive predictive value: 52%; negative predictive value: 96.8%).[6] The KFSI is usually used in the context of an in-depth psychological interview of the parent and may, therefore, not be appropriate for use as a general screening in a busy office.

The Hawaii Risk Indicators Screening Tool[7] was developed from a study of home visits of at-risk families. This tool was designed to be used as part of a medical record review or an in-depth interview with parents.[7] It is composed of 15 parental factors that make a child at high risk for abuse or neglect. The risk factors include parental depression, inadequate income or unemployment, lack of a phone, unstable housing, history of psychiatric care or substance abuse, inadequate prenatal care, history of abortions in the past or attempted abortion with the current child, or less than a high school education.[7]

For a more practical approach, Table 16–2 offers some examples of ways to screen different family members for child abuse. Providers may ask parents general questions about their perception of the child's safety at school or in day care or about any behavioral changes exhibited by the child.[8] Young children may be observed playing, although this is often beyond the scope of a primary care or emergency department clinician. Children who play violent games or act out by hurting someone else may be at high risk for victimization. Verbal children may be asked general questions about their daily life to assess for presence of neglect or asked specific questions about areas of pain. In private, a child may be asked about the presence of violence in the household.

Any suspicion of child abuse or neglect based on any screening test by the clinician warrants a careful physical examination and possibly referral to an expert in treating children who are victims of abuse, if available. Most states

Table 16–2 Tips for Child Abuse Screening in Practice

Who to Screen	Methods of Screening
Parents	General questions about child's safety at home, day care, or school and any behavior changes.
Preverbal or preschool children	Observation of interaction between parent and child. Observation of child's behavior. Any concerns, should refer to specialist.
School-age children	General questions about daily life, support at home, any questionable injuries, inappropriate touching.

Source: Adapted from Stanford School of Medicine, Child abuse resource Web site. www.childabuse.stanford.edu. Accessed September 15, 2009.

mandate that healthcare providers report any suspicion of child abuse (Chapter 4). Clinicians may be reluctant to diagnose child abuse because of lack of confidence in their own ability to make the diagnosis abuse or the potentially negative impact on their relationship with the family. In addition, some providers may find mandated reporting a barrier to diagnosing possible abuse.[9]

Children with behavioral or psychiatric disabilities are at higher risk of child abuse. Therefore,clinicians should be particularly vigilant in assessing for victimization in these children.[10] During an office visit with a child who has behavioral or psychiatric conditions, the clinician should ask the parents specifically about possible abuse and parental stress. A clinician may say something like "Many parents find taking care of a child who has your child's condition very frustrating. How do you deal with your frustration?" In addition, parental alcohol or drug abuse may increase the risk of child abuse and should trigger persistent inquiry. The presence of intimate partner violence (IPV) also often increases the risk of child abuse.

SCREENING FOR INTIMATE PARTNER VIOLENCE

During the last two decades the medical community has increasingly viewed IPV as an important health-related condition and not as a private issue. Recognition that IPV has tremendous impact on health has led to efforts to identify and assist patients who are victims of IPV. Because women comprise most IPV victims and incur the most serious IPV-related injuries,[10-12] most major medical organizations in the United States (including the American Medical Association, the American Academy of Family Physicians, the American College of Obstetricians & Gynecologists, and the American College of Emergency Physicians) recommend that clinicians routinely ask all their adult female patients about IPV exposure.[13-16] Additionally, the Joint Commission on Accreditation of Healthcare Organizations requires hospitals to have protocols for identifying and assisting victims of IPV to receive accreditation.[17] Currently, no national guidelines address IPV victimization in men.[18]

There is controversy over the lack of evidence to support such wide-scale IPV inquiry. As noted earlier, in 2004, the USPSTF issued a statement concluding that insufficient evidence existed to recommend for or against IPV screening.[2,19] This statement produced a strong response from the health care and advocacy communities.[20-23] Specifically, these constituencies argued that the USPSTF had assessed IPV screening as a screening test rather than as a behavioral assessment and counseling service and had placed too stringent a requirement for evidence linking IPV screening to reduced morbidity and/or mortality.[20,23]

A recently published randomized trial of IPV screening that showed no difference in outcomes between the screened and nonscreened groups has further fueled the debate about routine screening.[24] Although this study attempted to assess the difference between women who received IPV screening and those who did not, in reality all women in the trial were asked about IPV via validated written screening instruments. The only difference between the two groups was that the intervention arm included an additional in-person screening session before the initial clinical encounter. Both groups were screened immediately after this encounter and at regular follow-up intervals, and ultimately both groups demonstrated a decrease in reported IPV.

Qualitative research supports the important role that brief conversations with healthcare providers about IPV can play in making abused women feel supported and encouraged to seek help and/or change their situations.[25,26] The Transtheoretical Model of Behavioral Change as it applies to IPV victimization underscores the efficacy of such ongoing discussions in reducing violence victimization.[27] Using this model of motivational interviewing can help clinicians be patient centered in their counseling efforts of IPV victims.

Screening for IPV may be an intervention in and of itself, but further research is needed to prove this. Clinicians should continue to screen all their adult female patients for partner abuse because the prevalence and health effects of IPV warrant routine inquiry.[28,29] Repeated routine screening in primary care also may reduce the stigma of talking about IPV and may empower women to disclose their abuse history.

When to Screen

Patients with a history of IPV are frequently encountered in all medical specialties. One large study of partner abuse demonstrated that 26% of women in primary care practices, 35% of obstetrics/gynecology patients, and 41% of women presenting to emergency departments reported victimization by an intimate partner at some time in their lives.[30] Screening for IPV is acceptable to female patients.[31,32] Many women do not disclose IPV at the first screen but may be more likely to disclose with repeated screening.[33,34] Therefore, clinicians should screen periodically even when the initial screen was negative. For instance, primary care clinicians may want to screen at well exams, and emergency department physicians or hospitalists may want to screen at intake interviews. Only a minority (approximately 10%) of healthcare providers routinely screen their female patients for partner abuse.[35,36]

How to Screen

There are many available screening tools that have been designed to capture physical, sexual, and/or emotional abuse exposure.[2,37] These tools also serve as templates for the types of behaviorally specific IPV inquiry that may be adopted in clinical practice. Asking about specific acts of violence (e.g., hitting, kicking, pushing) may lead to fewer false-negative responses and may be a useful approach to IPV screening.[38-40] Additionally, clarifying the relationship of the abuser to the patient may reduce false-positive screening results (e.g., "Has your boyfriend hit, kicked, or pushed you?").[41]

IPV screening should be done in a safe, private setting. Screening modalities other than in-person interviews (e.g., computer-based or written questionnaires) may be employed in the patient care setting without compromising detection of IPV and may, in fact, be preferred by some patients.[42-44] When in-person interviews are conducted, nobody else, including children, should be present. Providers should be aware that sometimes interpreters may have personal ties to the patient and therefore could potentially compromise open communication about interpersonal violence. If such concerns arise, relying on hospital or clinic translators or telephone interpreting services would be prudent.

There are many different ways to screen for IPV in clinical practice. No one method has been proven to be superior to another.

Experts recommend that clinicians:

1. Begin IPV screening with a general statement about the prevalence of violence in our society to normalize the questions. For example: "Because violence is so common in our society, I ask all of my patients about violence in their lives."
2. Follow with an open-ended question about partner abuse exposure. For example: "Do you feel safe in your current relationship?" or "Do you feel safe at home?"
3. Ask about specific types of abuse. For example: "Does your partner/husband/boyfriend ever hit, kick, punch, threaten, or try to make you do things you don't want to do? Does your partner/husband/boyfriend ever force you to do something sexually that you do not want to do?"[37]

Such inquiry can take just a few minutes. If a clinician suspects abuse, but the patient does not disclose it during IPV screening, the clinician should inform the patient of this concern in a gentle, nonjudgmental manner. Such an approach might be: "I am concerned that someone may be hurting you at home and I would like to check in with you in a few weeks" or "I am concerned that your injuries do not fit the situation you described and I would like to see you again soon." At subsequent visits, the provider should address IPV as part of the patient's ongoing problem list. Many victims of IPV will not disclose their violent situations during a onetime clinical encounter.[32,45]

Like many patients confronting major decisions affecting their well-being, IPV victims exhibit varying degrees of insight and action regarding their abusive situations. As mentioned earlier, the Stages of Change model is a helpful construct for healthcare providers to use when trying to understand their interactions with abused women.[27] Victims in the precontemplation phase (the first phase of the model) may not recognize their partners' behavior as abusive, may minimize the seriousness of the abuse, or may simply feel hopeless about any benefits of disclosure.[27,46,47] Victims in the contemplation stage may be thinking about leaving the abusive situation but do not have a specific plan. Therefore, the process of screening for abuse may be a therapeutic modality in itself, as well as a mode of patient education about IPV, although this has not been proven yet.

In addition to being in denial about their circumstances, patients may withhold information about abuse out of shame, fear of repercussions, or concerns about confidentiality.[25,26,32,48] By directly addressing privacy issues at the beginning of IPV screening, clinicians can foster an environment in which abused women feel comfortable discussing this issue. Although beyond the scope of this chapter, the overwhelming majority of states do not require mandatory reporting of IPV to law enforcement authorities unless injury has been inflicted with a gun or a knife (exceptions include California, Colorado, and Kentucky).[49] Before any screening or discussion of partner abuse occurs, clinicians should discuss confidentiality issues with their patients.

Intimate Partner Violence Screening in Pediatrics

In 1998, the American Academy of Pediatrics (AAP) recommended IPV screening of female caretakers during their children's well-child visits.[50] The AAP considers questions about violence as part of anticipatory guidance counseling within a pediatric visit. Although screening instruments established for adult patient care settings may be applied,[41] it is important to remember that screening in the pediatric setting at times confers additional risks regarding patient confidentiality and child well-being. Logistically, it may be difficult to ask for privacy to conduct IPV screening among female caregivers. (For example, who will supervise the children while mothers are being screened?) Nonetheless, women should be asked about IPV outside the earshot of children who are beyond toddler age.[51] For instance, children may be taken out of the exam room with a nurse under the pretense of doing a vision test or getting a sticker or a toy. Screening in front of older children allows the possibility that the abuser may learn of the discussion and retaliate against the mother and/or her children. Lastly, deferring documentation of IPV-related discussions in the chart (i.e., not writing anything down about the visit) may be necessary because abusers could have access (as legal guardians) to a child's medical record.

SCREENING FOR ELDER ABUSE

Although the elderly are two to three times more likely to visit a healthcare facility than are young people, elder abuse is frequently not recognized.[52] Most cases are identified by provider screening in the healthcare setting or by third-party observers (i.e., case workers, family members, or other health professionals) and not by self-disclosure.[52] Many victims may not disclose violence because of concerns over confidentiality (i.e., that their abuser might learn of their disclosure and retaliate). In addition, some older adults may have cognitive impairments that preclude an accurate description of their abuse.[52]

Elders should be screened periodically at well visits and in any case of injury. Many screening tools are available. However, most instruments are cumbersome and not validated. There is a paucity of research into screening tools and screening methods, likely because of the multiple different types of abuse possible. Elders may be victims of physical violence, psychological violence, neglect, and financial abuse. Elders also may experience self-neglect, where they do not take care of their own basic needs (see Chapter 13 on elder abuse). An ideal screening test for the clinical setting would need to assess all of these facets of abuse and be brief, accurate, and easy to administer. Fulmer et al reviewed all available screening tools and recommended using the Elder Assessment Instrument (EAI), the Conflict Tactics Scale (CTS), or the Brief Abuse Screen for the Elderly (BASE).[52] Another commonly employed screening tool is the shortened version of the Hwalek-Sengstock Elder Abuse Screening Test (H-S/EAST). The Elder Assessment Instrument is a 42-item checklist completed by a clinician.[53] Administration of this instrument requires training, but it is suitable for use in a clinic setting as well as in a home-based assessment. The EAI provides a comprehensive evaluation of physical and psychological abuse, as well as neglect and exploitation, and is available in Spanish.[53] The length of the instrument could be a barrier for busy clinicians, however, and may limit its usefulness in clinical encounters.

The CTS is another comprehensive screening instrument that may be employed in both clinic encounters and in the home.[54] Developed in 1979 at the Family Research Laboratory at the University of New Hampshire, it has been studied extensively over the past 30 years and validated for detecting intrafamily violence. However, the CTS does not measure psychological violence and is not specific to elders.[54] It includes a 19-item self-administered questionnaire and is also available in Spanish. The major limitation of the CTS in a busy clinical practice is its length.

The BASE is a five-question survey completed by trained personnel concerning their opinion about whether a patient may be a victim of abuse, the identity of the abuser, and the urgency of the situation.[55] This screen has been validated and has inter-evaluator reliability of 86–90%.[55] However, this screen does not assess for indicators of neglect,[52] nor has it been tested in a busy clinical setting. The BASE shows promise because of its brevity and accuracy, but it does not directly ask the potential victim any questions.

The shortened version of the H-S/EAST includes six questions to ask the potential victim that are very similar to those included in the AMA's recommendation on screening for elder abuse.[56] This screen shows promise as a short, easy-to-use screen in a busy clinical practice.[57] The six questions are as follows:

1. Are you afraid of anyone in your family?
2. Has anyone close to you tried to hurt or harm you recently?
3. Has anyone close to you called you names or put you down or made you feel bad recently?
4. Does someone in your family make you stay in bed or tell you that you are sick when you know you aren't?
5. Has anyone forced you to do things you didn't want to?
6. Has anyone taken things that belong to you without your okay?

These six questions are easy to use and fast. However, they have not been validated in diverse populations and do not screen for self-neglect.

Further revision of the shortened H-S/EAST[58] expanded the screen to include 12 questions that cover four areas: vulnerability, dependence, dejection, and coercion. This expanded instrument is more comprehensive than the short version of the H-S/EAST and includes measures of self-neglect. It still needs to be validated in diverse populations and tested in a busy clinical practice.

None of the instruments just described is clearly superior to any other. Each has strengths and weaknesses, and none has been shown to affect outcomes (ending of the abuse). Ultimately, many clinicians may choose to use indirect questions to determine the presence of abuse or neglect. Questions that may help the clinician understand an older adult's daily life, involvement with family and friends, and the ability to take care of oneself may uncover evidence of abuse. Recommendations from the National Guidelines Clearinghouse include a suggestion for the clinician to ask general questions of the older adult (such as, "How are things at home?"; "Do you feel safe at home?") before using a specific screening instrument.[59]

Table 16–3 Helpful Web Sites for Clinicians Regarding Elder Abuse Screening

MedAmerica Insurance Company	www.MedAmericaLTC.com
	• Single-page tool for clinicians
Maine Partners for Elder Protection	http://www.umaine.edu/mainecenteronaging/mepep.htm
	• Manual describing a screening protocol in primary care office practices
Elder Response Team: Family Violence Task Force	http://www.elderresponseteam.org/Elder%20Abuse%20 Screening.htm
	• Screening quizzes for patients or caregivers to identify elders at high risk of abuse or fraud

Several online resources may be useful for the clinician. MedAmerica Insurance Company developed a single-page elder abuse assessment and management tool that is available online.[60] This tool may be helpful to clinicians because it includes a concise assessment and management guidelines for the identification of elder mistreatment. The Maine Partners for Elder Protection also developed a screening protocol for physicians.[61] This clinical guideline recommends that all patients older than 60 years should be screened at least annually at a nonurgent office visit. The protocol has been pilot-tested in a number of different clinical settings. Various members of the healthcare team may administer the six-question screen that include questions about being afraid at home, being forced to do things the elder does not want to do, and being prevented from using the telephone.[61] Other helpful Web sites are listed in Table 16–3.

CONCLUSION

All types of family violence are common in our society. Clinicians should think about abuse in all clinical situations and screen children, women, and elders vigilantly in an effort to improve the safety of potential victims.

REFERENCES

1. Gordis L. *Epidemiology*. 3rd ed. Philadelphia, PA: WB Saunders; 2004.
2. Nelson HD, Nygren P, McInerney Y, Klein J. Screening women and elderly adults for family and intimate partner violence: a review of the evidence for the US Preventive Services Task Force. *Ann Intern Med.* 2004;140(5):387–396.
3. Tjaden P, Thoennes N. *Full Report of the Prevalence, Incidence, and Consequences of Violence Against Women: Findings from the National Violence Against Women Survey.* Washington, DC: National Institute of Justice and Centers for Disease Control and Prevention; 2000.

4. Nygren P, Nelson HD, Klein J. Screening children for family violence: a review of the evidence for the US Preventive Services Task Force. *Ann Fam Med.* 2004;2(2):161-169.

5. Appendix 3: Screening Instruments. Health Services/Technology Assessment Screening (HSTAT) for family and intimate partner violence. National Library of Science Web site. http://www.ncbi.nlm.nih.gov/books/bv.fcgi?indexed=google &rid=hstat3.section.35848. Accessed September 15. 2009.

6. Korfmacher J. The Kempe Family Stress Inventory: a review. *Child Abuse Negl.* 2000;24(1):129-140.

7. Duggan A, Windham A, McFarlane E, et al. Hawaii's healthy start program of home visiting for at-risk families: evaluation of family identification, family engagement, and service delivery. *Pediatrics.* 2000;105:250-259.

8. Child abuse resource. Stanford School of Medicine Web site. http://www.childabuse. stanford.edu. Accessed September 15, 2009.

9. Flaherty EG, Sege R. Barriers to physician identification and reporting of child abuse. *Pediatr Ann North Am.* 2005;34(5):349-356.

10. Jaudes PK, Mackey-Bilaver L. Do chronic conditions increase young children's risk of being mistreated? *Child Abuse Negl.* 2008;32:671-681.

11. Tjaden P, Thoennes N. *Extent, Nature and Consequences of Intimate Partner Violence: Findings from the National Violence Against Women Survey.* Washington, DC: National Institute of Justice and Centers for Disease Control and Prevention; 2000.

12. Centers for Disease Control and Prevention. Adverse health conditions and health risk behaviors associated with intimate partner violence—United States 2005. *MMWR.* 2008;57:113-117.

13. *National Advisory Council on Violence and Abuse: Policy Compendium.* AMA Online Report, Chicago, IL; 2008. American Medical Association Web site. http:// www. ama-assn.org/ama1/pub/upload/mm/386/vio_policy_comp.pdf. Accessed September 13, 2010.

14. American Academy of Family Physicians. *Policy on Family and Intimate Partner Violence and Abuse.* Leawood, KS: AAFP; 2004. AAFP Web site. http://www.aafp. org/online/en/home/policy/policies/f/familyandintimatepartner-violenceandabuse. html. Accessed September 13, 2010.

15. American College of Obstetrics and Gynecology. *Special Issues in Women's Health: Intimate Partner Violence and Domestic Violence.* Washington, DC: ACOG; 2005.

16. American College of Emergency Physicians. *Policy on Domestic Family Violence.* Irving, TX: ACEP; 2007. Available at http://www.acep.org/practres.aspx?id=29184.

17. Family Violence Prevention Fund: JCAHO Additional Standards for Victims of Abuse Standard PC.3.10. San Francisco, CA: FVPF; 2008. Available at http:// endabuse.org/ programs/printable/display.php3?DocID=266.

18. Kimberg LS. Addressing intimate partner violence in male patients: a review and introduction of pilot guidelines. *J Gen Intern Med.* 2008;23:2071-2078.

19. US Preventive Services Task Force. Screening for family and intimate partner violence: recommendation statement. *Ann Intern Med.* 2004;140:382-386.

20. American Medical Association. *Report 7 of the Council on Scientific Affairs: Diagnosis and Management of Family Violence.* Chicago, IL: AMA Online Report; 2005. Available at http://www.ama-assn.org/ama/pub/category/15248.html.

21. Lachs MS. Screening for family violence: what's an evidence-based doctor to do? *Ann Intern Med.* 2004;140:399-400.

22. Spangaro J, Zwi AB, Poulos R. The elusive search for definitive evidence on routine screening for intimate partner violence. *Trauma Violence Abuse.* 2009;10: 55–68.

23. Chamberlain L. *The USPSTF Recommendation on Intimate Partner Violence: What We Can Learn from It and What Can We Do About It.* San Francisco, CA: Family Violence Prevention Fund; 2005.

24. MacMillan HL, Wathen NC, Jamieson E, et al. Screening for intimate partner violence in health care settings: a randomized trial. *JAMA.* 2009;302:493–501.

25. Feder GS, Hutson M, Ramsay J, Taket AR. Women exposed to intimate partner violence: expectations and experiences when they encounter health care professionals: a meta-analysis of qualitative studies. *Arch Intern Med.* 2006;166:22–37.

26. McCauley J, Yurk RA, Jenckes JW, Ford DE. Inside "Pandora's box": abused women's experiences with clinicians and health services. *J Gen Intern Med.* 1998;13:549–555.

27. Zink T, Elder N, Jacobson J, Klostermann B. Medical management of intimate partner violence considering the stages of change: precontemplation and contemplation. *Ann Fam Med.* 2004;2: 231–239.

28. Gerber MR, Wittenberg E, Ganz ML, Williams CM, McCloskey LA. Intimate partner violence exposure and change in women's physical symptoms over time. *J Gen Intern.* 2008;23:64–69.

29. Bonomi AE, Thompson RS, Anderson M, et al. Intimate partner violence and women's physical, mental, and social functioning. *Am J Prev Med.* 2006;30:458–466.

30. McCloskey LA, Lichter E, Ganz ML, et al. Intimate partner violence and patient screening across medical specialties. *Acad Emerg Med.* 2005;12:712–722.

31. Friedman LS, Samet JH, Roberts MS, Hudlin M, Hans P. Inquiry about victimization experiences: a survey of patient preferences and physician practices. *Arch Intern Med.* 1992;152:1186–1190.

32. Renker PR, Tonkin P. Women's views of prenatal violence screening: acceptability and confidentiality issues. *Obstet Gynecol.* 2006;107:348–354.

33. McFarlane J, Parker B, Soeken K, Bullock MS. Assessing for abuse during pregnancy: severity and frequency of injuries and associated entry into prenatal care. *JAMA.* 1992;267:3176–3178.

34. Bullock L, Bloom T, Davis J, Kilburn E, Curry MA. Abuse disclosure in privately and medicaid-funded pregnant women. *J Midwifery Womens Health.* 2006;51:361–369.

35. Rodriguez MA, Bauer HM, McLoughlin E, Grumbach K. Screening and intervention for intimate partner abuse: practices and attitudes of primary care physicians. *JAMA.* 1999;282:468–474.

36. Elliott L, Nerney M, Jones T, Friedmann PD. Barriers to screening for domestic violence. *J Gen Intern Med.* 2002;17:112–116.

37. Phelan MB. Screening for intimate partner violence in medical settings. *Trauma Violence Abuse.* 2007;8:199–213.

38. Reichenheim ME, Moraes CL. Comparison between the abuse assessment screen and the revised conflict tactics scales for measuring physical violence during pregnancy. *J Epidemiol Community Health.* 2004;58:523–527.

39. Glander SS, Moore ML, Michielutte R, Parsons LH. The prevalence of domestic violence among women seeking abortion. *Obstet Gynecol.* 1998;91:1002–1006.

40. Peralta, RL, Fleming MF. Screening for intimate partner violence in a primary care setting: the validity of "feeling safe at home" and prevalence results. *J Am Board Fam Pract.* 2003;16:525–532.

41. Holtrop TG, Fischer H, Gray SM, Barry K, Bryant T, Du W. Screening for domestic violence in a general pediatric clinic: be prepared. *Pediatrics.* 2004;114:1253–1257.

42. Ahmad F, Hogg-Johnson S, Stewart DE, Skinner HA, Glazier RH, Levinson W. Computer-assisted screening for intimate partner violence and control: a randomized trial. *Ann Intern Med.* 2009;151:93–102.

43. MacMillan HL, Wathen CN, Jamieson E, et al.; McMaster Violence Against Women Research Group. Approaches to screening for intimate partner violence in health care settings: a randomized trial. *JAMA.* 2006;296:530–536.

44. Canterino JC, VanHorn LG, Harrigan JT, Ananth CV, Vintzileos AM. Domestic abuse in pregnancy: a comparison of a self-completed domestic abuse questionnaire with a directed interview. *Am J Obstet Gynecol.* 1999;181:1049–1051.

45. Kothari CL, Rhodes KV. Missed opportunities: emergency department visits by police-identified victims of intimate partner violence. *Ann Emerg Med.* 2006;47:190–199.

46. Burke JG, Gielen AC, McDonnell KA, O'Campo P, Maman S. The process of ending abuse in intimate relationships: a qualitative exploration of the transtheoretical model. *Violence Against Women.* 2001;7:1144–1163.

47. Frasier PY, Slatt L, Kowlowitz V, Glowa PT. Using the stages of change model to counsel victims of intimate partner violence. *Patient Educ Couns.* 2001;43:211–217.

48. Rodriguez MA, Sheldon WR, Bauer HM, Perez-Stable EJ. The factors associated with disclosure of intimate partner abuse to clinicians. *J Fam Pract.* 2001;50: 338–344.

49. Family Violence Prevention Fund. *State Codes on Intimate Partner Violence Victimization Reporting Requirements for Health Care Providers.* San Francisco, CA: FVPF; 2002. Available at http://www.endabuse.org/health/mandatoryreporting/tables1.pdf.

50. Committee on Child Abuse and Neglect, American Academy of Pediatrics. The role of the pediatrician in recognizing and intervening on behalf of abused women. *Pediatrics.* 1998;101:1091–1092.

51. Zink T. Should children be in the room when the mother is screened for partner violence? *J Fam Pract.* 2000;49:130–136.

52. Fulmer T, Guadagno L, Dyer CB, Connolly MT. Progress in elder abuse screening and assessment instruments. *J Am Geriatr Soc.* 2004;52:297–304.

53. Fulmer T, Street S, Carr K. Abuse of the elderly: screening and detection. *J Emerg Nurs.* 1984;10:131–140.

54. Straus MA. Measuring intrafamily conflict and violence. The Conflict Tactics Scale(CTS)—Form A. *J Marriage Fam.* 1979;41:75–88.

55. Reis M, Nahmiash D. Validation of the indicators of abuse (IOA) screen. *Gerontologist.* 1998;38(4):471–480.

56. AMA's Diagnostic and Treatment Guidelines on Elder Abuse and Neglect (1992).

57. Schofield MJ, Reynolds R, Mishra GD, Powers JR, Dobson AJ. Screening for vulnerability to abuse among older women: women's health Australia study. *J Appl Gerontol.* 2002;21:24–39.

58. Schofield MJ, Mishra GD. Validity of self-report screening scale for elder abuse: women's health Australia study. *Gerontologist.* 2003;43:110–120.

59. Daly JM. Elder abuse prevention. Iowa City (IA): University of Iowa Gerontological Nursing Interventions Research Center, Research Dissemination Core; 2004 Dec. 68 p. [111 references]. Available at http://www.guideline.gov/summary/summary. aspx?ss=15 &doc_id=6829&nbr=4196. Accessed September 15, 2009.

60. Bomba PA. Use of a single page elder abuse assessment and management tool: a practical clinician's approach to identifying elder mistreatment. *J Gerontol Soc Work.* 2006;46:103–122.

61. University of Maine Center on Aging. Elder abuse screening protocol for physicians: lessons learned from the Maine Partners for Elder Protection Pilot Project, version 5/2007. University of Maine Web site. http://www.umaine.edu/ mainecenteronaging/documents/elderabusescreeningmanual.pdf. Accessed September 15, 2009.

Chapter 17

The Clinical Encounter

Sarina Schrager, MD, MS

CASE EXAMPLE

A 25-year-old white female whom you have never met before presents with an asthma exacerbation. While doing a lung exam, you notice ecchymoses on her upper arms and back. You order a nebulizer treatment. While she is getting her treatment, you review her chart. She has been seen multiple times in the emergency department and at the urgent care clinic for various orthopaedic complaints, including knee pain, ankle sprain, and wrist pain, and also for head injury. Multiple clinicians document that they screened her for intimate partner violence (IPV), but she denies it. She has also been seen multiple times by one of your partners for chronic abdominal pain. That workup was negative. Once the nebulizer treatment is over and her breathing is improved, you return to the room and tell her that you noticed the bruising on her arms and back. You also tell her that it is common for someone with her history (chronic pain, multiple injuries) to be a victim of violence. You ask her if someone is hurting her at home.

The patient starts to cry and admits that her husband drinks alcohol and that when he drinks he gets angry if she has not cleaned up after the kids or doesn't have dinner ready. And he hits her. He is always very sorry afterwards and promises that it will never happen again. She now thinks that he is not going to stop, because it always happens again. No matter how careful she is and how hard she works, he always finds something about which to be angry. The violence has escalated and is occurring more frequently. He lost his job and is home all the time, drinking a lot. She has thought about leaving, but she doesn't have a job and has three children younger than 5 years. She is afraid that if she leaves, she will not be able to support herself and her children. She doesn't think that she has anywhere to go. She has not told anyone else about the violence before now. She is embarrassed to tell her family because they told her not to marry him in the first place. Her husband is in the waiting room, and she is scared that he will find out that she told you about the violence.

CASE DISCUSSION

This is a typical scenario in which a woman has denied being abused over and over to health professionals but is finally ready to admit it. In this case, it is especially important to tell the patient that the abuse is not her fault, that she doesn't deserve to be treated that way, and that there are people who can help her.

INTRODUCTION

With the recommendations for universal screening for IPV in healthcare settings, many healthcare practitioners will be faced with a situation where a woman* says "yes" to the screening questions. The answer "yes" to a screening question may provoke anxiety in the practitioner. S/he may feel ill equipped to handle the situation, may worry that the visit will take longer than a typical office visit, and, in some states, may be concerned about mandatory reporting laws (see Chapter 21). In many ways, a patient who is a victim of IPV challenges the clinician–patient relationship. This relationship is important to help end the abuse. This chapter describes practical suggestions for clinicians to use to manage these situations.

Supportive Response

Many women do not disclose that they are in a violent relationship. The factors that impact whether a woman discloses abuse to the clinician are complicated. Sensitivity of screening (i.e., privacy, unhurried method, compassionate language) is very important to encourage disclosure.[1] Many women may feel embarrassed about the abuse or are afraid that their partner will discover that they talked to a clinician about the abuse, and, therefore, they will not disclose. In violent relationships, the abuser often

---

*Since 85% of all victims of IPV are female,[9] this chapter considers the victims as women and uses the pronoun *she* when describing victims. The same suggestions would be appropriate for a male victim.

threatens the victim with an escalation of violence in response to disclosure. Providing a safe, supportive, and private atmosphere for discussion will encourage the victim to disclose the abuse. Even so, as illustrated above, many women will be asked multiple times by multiple providers before they finally disclose the violence in their relationships. It is sometimes unclear how multiple factors work together to enable a woman to admit that she is in a violent relationship. In this case, the patient probably did not feel well and was ready to admit that the relationship was not going to change and the violence was not going to end. It is important for clinicians to always be ready for a "yes" response, because often it will be a surprise, coming after frequent "nos."

Other factors that impact on whether a woman will disclose an experience of violence include the presence of her children at the visit or the time constraints of the clinician. Whether or not to screen for violence in front of children will depend on the age of the children.[2] If a woman comes to a visit with her partner (the abuser), obviously she will be unable to inform the clinician about any abuse. In that situation, any effort to separate the victim from the abuser will be helpful to enable the clinician to obtain the truth. In some practices, the patient will be asked to give a urine sample in a woman's bathroom or do something in another private place in order to get her alone. Many abusers, though, will be suspicious of attempts by healthcare professionals to separate them from the victim, so this attempt must be done with caution to avoid an escalation of violence after the visit. If the woman's partner refuses to leave, clinicians should have a high suspicion of abuse and should make a note about it in the chart so they can follow up at another scheduled visit.

Clinicians often do not ask about abuse because they are afraid of getting a "yes" response. However, violence is so common that it is nearly impossible to avoid. In a survey of physicians in Canada, over 80% of the 328 surveyed had experienced a disclosure of IPV within the last year.[3] Clinicians may hear about abuse in response to a general screening question or while investigating an injury. Being educated about the issue and proactive in learning adequate responses to a "yes" answer will make clinicians more comfortable in the situation. Regardless of comfort level, the discussion of abuse is not one that can take place adequately in a standard 15-minute office visit. Consequently, clinicians may need help from other health professionals (e.g., nurses, social workers, therapists) in managing the situation. However, the clinician, in this case, is the "first responder" to the victim and must be trained to react appropriately to the disclosure. The first response may set the stage for the victim's comfort in discussing her situation and her experience with the health profession as a whole. Interviews with 27 women who were victims of IPV found that unhelpful interactions with the health professional (i.e., interactions that were negative but did not cause any harm) were associated with emotional distress and a sense of alienation from the healthcare system at large.[4] In this particular study, most of the unhelpful interactions occurred in the emergency department as opposed to a primary care office.

Clinicians should stop what they are doing, make eye contact, and speak directly to a patient who discloses that she is in an abusive relationship. Empathy and compassion are important in a first response to the disclosure. Table 17-1 provides an example of some ways to respond immediately. The clinician should be explicit in saying that the abuse is not the victim's fault, that it is wrong for any person to hurt another, and should express genuine concern for the victim's well-being. The clinician should not act surprised, because many women feel they are the only ones who have experienced violence. Validating her experience by using nonjudgmental language and behavior will help make her feel that the clinician is a safe person with whom to talk to and may mitigate some potential embarrassment. Interviews with 32 women who were in shelters or support groups for violence found that women had four clear expectations from clinicians after disclosure of abuse.[5] Women wanted their clinician to (1) affirm that the abuse really happened, (2) be knowledgeable about local IPV resources and inform the patient about them, (3) educate the victims about the consequences of abuse on themselves and their children, and (4) document any injuries in the medical record. A meta-analysis of studies examining what women wanted from clinicians in response to a disclosure of violence also included a respect for each woman's timeline and no pressure to talk about the abuse, to leave, or to prosecute the abuser.[6] This meta-analysis of 29 studies also found that women wanted clinicians to be nonjudgmental and to realize that every situation is unique.[6] Implicit in these expectations is the idea that each woman will make decisions about whether to stay in the relationship differently. In summary, women want the clinician to understand the complexity of a violent relationship and to meet them where they are in the continuum of deciding what to do.

Table 17-1 Examples of What to Say When Your Patient Discloses Abuse

I believe you. That must be a horrible experience.

I'm sorry that you have to experience that. I would like to help.

The abuse is not your fault. It is wrong for one person to hurt another person.

You didn't do anything to deserve to be treated this way.

I'm glad you told me. Let's think about ways to get this behavior to stop.

Unfortunately, you are not alone. Many of my patients have experienced abuse.

I am worried about your safety.

RISK ASSESSMENT

After validating the patient's experience and expressing concern about her safety, an assessment of immediate danger is imperative. If the abuser is at the office and the victim does not want to leave with him due to concerns about her immediate safety, the clinician may have to call the police (with the consent of the victim). In the case example, the patient needs to decide whether to go home with her partner, and the clinician needs to be assured of her immediate safety. Factors that affect acuity of abuse include the abuser's previous use of force, alcohol or drug use, and availability of weapons in the home.[2] Many women may not realize that they are in imminent danger. A case-control study found that more than half of the victims of a completed or attempted homicide did not think that they were in danger.[7] If an abuser has access to sharp knives, firearms, or other weapons, the risk of lethal violence increases. Additionally, if the abuser has used severe force in the past or has threatened to do so or is known to abuse alcohol or drugs, the victim's risk increases.[8] Another high-risk situation is one in which the abuser has stalked the victim or has held her hostage.[2] Clinicians also should ask about any recent escalation in threats or violence. In these situations, the clinician may advocate for the victim to leave the situation and look for a safe place to stay. In the absence of immediate danger, the discussion turns to a more long-term approach to safety.

The goal of the encounter is to support the victim while trying to keep her and her children safe. The clinician may be faced with a dilemma if she or he feels the victim is not safe but the victim does not agree. The clinician should try to empower the victim to remain in control of her situation and be careful not to make decisions for her. The clinician should not try to force a woman to leave an abusive situation if she is not ready. The clinician may adversely affect the doctor–patient relationship if s/he pressures a woman to do something s/he is not ready to do. The victim also may face an escalation of abuse related to any discussion of leaving.

If a woman admits to having a current injury from a violent partner, the clinician should document the injury with photographs and a detailed description of how the injury occurred. Specific descriptions of findings and mechanism of injury should be included in a confidential note in the patient's chart. Some paper charts have a separate folder for confidential notes about psychiatric or substance abuse issues. Discussions of violence should be kept in these special files. Some electronic medical record programs enable password-protected subcharts to be kept. For example, in the case described here, the clinician should describe the ecchymoses on the patient's back and arms in detail or take a photograph with her consent. The clinician also should assess the victim for any thoughts of suicide or homicide and refer her appropriately.[2] Suicidal thoughts may necessitate a psychological consultation. Homicidal thoughts (i.e., thoughts or plans to kill the abuser) should be assessed for seriousness, and consultation with a legal professional may be necessary. In some situations it may be necessary to call the police.

SAFETY PLAN

A safety plan for an abused individual can have several components. The first task is to plan how to stay safe in the home. A woman can think about where to go to stay away from her abuser. There may be rooms with doors that lock or places in the house that are more public where she may be safer. If she thinks it is safe, she may tell neighbors about the situation so they can call the police if they hear arguing or loud noises. She may want to stay out of rooms with potential weapons during an argument, such as the kitchen where there may be knives or places where any firearms may be hidden. She may want to think about staying between her abuser and the door so that she can possibly take her children and run away or out of the room if threatened.

The second part of a safety plan is to think about a time when the abuse gets so severe that she may want to leave the house, even for a few hours. In situations of immediate danger, the patient will not have time to think about what to take with her. Thus, she should plan ahead and pack a bag or backpack with some essential items that she will need if she leaves the house. Table 17–2 lists some items to include in an emergency bag. The victim should keep copies of important papers, such as her Social Security card and her children's birth certificates, along with cash, car keys, and important phone numbers (e.g., family, local violence hotline, shelters). She should hide the bag outside of the house in a safe place so that when she is

Table 17–2 What to Pack in an Emergency Bag

Cash	List of emergency phone numbers
Car keys	Directions to local shelter
Copies of identification for self and children (driver's license, Social Security card, birth certificates, health insurance cards)	Phone number for the National Domestic Violence Hotline, 1-800-799-SAFE
Nonperishable food (e.g., granola bars, dried fruit, nuts)	Disposable cell phone
Change of clothes for victim and children	Medication
Toiletries	Small toys for children

in immediate danger, she can just leave. She also should plan for what she will do with her children. She may want to go to a friend's house or a hotel. In some situations, going to a family member's house may not be safe because that may be the first place the abuser will look for her. If she goes to a shelter or finds another place to stay, she should keep her location secret so the abuser cannot find her. She should also choose a "code" word to be used with trusted neighbors, friends, or family members that denotes immediate danger and instructs them to call the police.

RESOURCES

Clinicians should know about the local resources available to help victims of violence. Most communities have 24-hour telephone hotlines that both clinicians and victims can call for information, support, or problem solving. Information is usually provided in a nondescript manner that will not arouse suspicion by the abuser. Some hotlines and shelters provide cards with information on them that are hidden in a lipstick container or a pillbox. Many communities also have safe, secret shelters in which women can stay with their children after they have left the abuser. Most shelters provide legal assistance to women who are trying to either file for divorce from the abuser or get a restraining order. Shelters have been successful in preventing further abuse as well.[9] Online resources such as the Family Violence Prevention Fund Web site (www.endabuse.org) also can be helpful for the victim and the healthcare practitioner. Clinicians can provide the victim with a private phone so that she can make contact with local or national support personnel (such as the National Domestic Violence Hotline, 1-800-799-SAFE) while still in the healthcare setting. There are also many support groups that can help the victim to feel less alone.

THE CLINICIAN–PATIENT RELATIONSHIP

If the victim discloses the abuse to the clinician, it is likely that she feels safe and comfortable in that particular healthcare environment. Most situations are subacute (not immediately life threatening) and are, therefore, often managed over a period of time. Modeling the treatment of IPV like the treatment of a chronic disease can be helpful for the clinician.[10] For instance, many women may not be considering leaving the relationship at the time of disclosure. Some, in fact, may be weeks, months, or even years away from actually leaving. Clinicians can become emotionally involved in seeing the patient leave the situation and are consequently disappointed and frustrated when the woman does not leave or leaves and returns. This frustration may be difficult to hide from the victim and may make her feel guilty that she "disappointed" the clinician, a safe person whom she trusts. Thus, a clinician would be well advised not to become emotionally involved in her leaving the abuser. This is a similar clinical situation to the care of a smoker or an alcoholic. The clinician should not get angry at the patient for not leaving when told. A goal for the relationship should be stopping the abuse, not necessarily leaving the abuser. By changing the focus, the clinician may be able to be more objective and helpful even when the victim does not leave. Table 17–3 includes some tips for clinicians. Clinicians should schedule frequent follow-up visits to check in with the patient and assess for any escalation of the violence, presence of a safety plan, use of any resources, and plans for the future.[2]

Women may not leave abusive situations for a variety of reasons, including financial issues, lack of a place to go, or having such low self-esteem that they do not feel that they can escape. A very real fear that many women have is that when they leave, the abuse will escalate. Women who are separated from the abuser are 25 times more likely to be assaulted by their abusers.[11] In addition, women who leave the abusive situation are most likely to be killed during the act of leaving. This is a very dangerous time for a victim. Up to a third of all women who leave will continue to be harmed by the abuser.[12] Women may leave multiple times and return before they finally decide to leave for good. The clinician needs to view the goal of leaving as a process, focus on small goals, schedule frequent follow-up visits to assess for immediate danger, provide support, and respect each woman's decision-making process. Specific interventions and support by the clinician will depend on where each woman is in the spectrum of deciding when or how to leave.[10] For instance, if she is not ready to leave, the clinician may provide information on the cycle of violence, how violence affects children's and women's health,

Table 17–3 Tips for Clinicians to Help them Avoid Frustration with Victims who do not Leave

Focus on stopping the violence, not on the victim leaving the abusive relationship.

View a violent relationship as a chronic disease and work on it slowly at frequent follow-up visits.

Respect the victim's timetable.

Understand the barriers to each woman's decision to leave or not and respect her decision.

Help the victim gain self-esteem by validating her actions, while at the same time being honest about your concern for her safety.

Remember that you may be one of the only people she feels comfortable talking with about the violence and try not to sabotage that relationship by being disappointed in her.

and some background about the wheel of power and control theory.[13] If a woman recognizes that she should leave and is beginning to think about it, the clinician may discuss in detail a safety plan and plans for her future life.

CONFIDENTIALITY ISSUES

All states have mandatory reporting laws for suspected child abuse, and most have laws for reporting suspected elder abuse. Some states have mandatory reporting laws regarding anyone who is a victim of domestic violence as well (see Chapter 21). Therefore, clinicians may need to be careful when discussing violence with their patients. Women need to know that if they disclose that their children are in danger, the clinician must legally call the state's child protective services bureau. Discussions of a woman's safety can be kept confidential, but discussion of a child's safety cannot. The clinician obviously does not want to do anything to potentially exacerbate the violence at home. The victim must be informed about mandatory reporting of child abuse. If the state is one of the few that requires mandated reporting for IPV, this would clearly be another barrier for some women to disclose. All clinicians should know their state's laws pertaining to family violence. A state-by-state listing is available at www.endabuse.org.

As noted above, keeping the medical records confidential is also critical.[2] For instance, if an abuser sees an itemized medical bill that includes injuries from the abuse, he may become angry and retaliate against the victim. In addition, employers or insurance companies who request records should not see discussions of abuse to prevent possible discrimination. Practices should discuss ways to keep such information confidential.

Another difficult situation may arise when the abuser is a patient at the same healthcare site. The provider must not share any information with him about his spouse. Working with perpetrators can be difficult, especially if you are not supposed to know that they are perpetrators (see Chapter 20). Clinicians may consider screening men for violent behavior. This might be a way to initiate a discussion of violence with the perpetrator that is objective and does not involve his victim, but it is not known how the perpetrator will respond. Alcohol use, depression, and history of childhood abuse are risk factors that have been associated with abuse by men in an intimate relationship.[14] However, as always, the clinician must be careful to not arouse suspicion that could potentially cause an escalation in the violence.

PATIENT EDUCATION

As part of the discussion after disclosure of violence, the clinician should provide information to the victim about the idea that the violence occurs as part of a cycle and about the effects of violence on children. As noted in Chapter 3, the cycle of violence describes a pattern of behavior that is common in a violent relationship. This pattern suggests that violence is rarely one isolated event; most violent relationships will continue in a cyclical pattern with an escalation of violence. Many women want to believe that "it won't happen again." Unfortunately, most will be incorrect. Women also should be aware of the impact on their children of witnessing violence (see Chapter 4). Children who witness violence are at a higher risk of developing psychological problems such as depression, anxiety, and posttraumatic stress disorder (PTSD). They also have higher rates of suicide attempts and drug and alcohol abuse and are at greater risk of being violent themselves.[15] Effects differ based on the age of the child. However, women may be reassured that some children do not have any long-term sequelae from witnessing abuse.[16] Some women who may not be able to leave for themselves may leave for the sake of their children.

PRACTICE SUPPORT

Healthcare offices can improve their response to victims of violence by training key personnel about screening for and management of IPV. In addition, posters, information cards, and buttons worn by clinicians or nurses all can communicate to the victim that the office is a safe place to disclose violence. It is not known what effect these public displays have on the abuser or the abuse itself. Many practices place posters in the women's bathrooms so that abusers will not see them. In some practices, individual clinicians and support staff complete extra training about violence so they can be a resource for the rest of the staff. Chart prompts can remind clinicians to screen for violence as well. The following factors are related to the comfort level of a practice in responding to victims of IPV: practices with on-site resources; adequate time available in an office visit; focused IPV training of clinicians and support staff; and a team approach to care. These make the setting more comfortable for staff in dealing with IPV victims.[16,17] Practices should consider inviting IPV professionals to educate staff on ways to improve their care of victims.

A small pilot study (41 women participated) demonstrated that intense follow-up of women who were victims of abuse increased their "safety-promoting" behaviors.[18] The primary care clinic intervention included a counseling session at the clinic and six follow-up phone calls over a 3-month period. The control group received printed educational materials about IPV and three follow-up phone calls to verify demographics.[18] In this study, the intervention group had fewer episodes of physical violence, less risk of lethal harm, and fewer symptoms of PTSD. This preliminary study shows promise as a way of empowering women to affect the type and frequency of abusive episodes. Primary care offices can use this model as an example of a structured approach to the care of victims of IPV.

REFERENCES

1. Falsetti SA. Screening and responding to family and intimate partner violence in the primary care setting. *Prim Care.* 2007;34:641–657.
2. National consensus guidelines on identifying and responding to domestic violence victimization in health care settings, 2004. Family Violence Prevention Fund Web site. www.endabuse.org.
3. Gutmanis I, Beynon C, Tutty L, Wathen CN, MacMillan HL. Factors influencing identification of and response to intimate partner violence: a survey of physicians and nurses. *BMC Public Health.* 2007;7:12.
4. Liebschutz J, Battaglia T, Finley E, Averbuch T. Disclosing intimate partner violence to health care clinicians—what a difference the setting makes: a qualitative study. *BMC Public Health.* 2008;8:229.
5. Zink T, Elder N, Jacobson J, Klostermann B. Medical management of intimate partner violence considering the stages of change: precontemplation and contemplation. *Ann Fam Med.* 2004;2(3):231–239.
6. Feder GS, Hutson M, Ramsay J, et al. Women exposed to intimate partner violence: expectations and experiences when they encounter health care professionals: a meta-analysis of qualitative studies. *Arch Intern Med.* 2006;166:22–37.
7. Campbell JC, Koziol-McLain J, Webster D, et al. *Research Results from a National Study of Intimate Partner Femicide: The Danger Assessment Instrument.* Washington, DC: National Institute of Justice; 2002.
8. Zolotor AJ, Denham AC, Weil A. Intimate partner violence. *Prim Care Clin Office Pract.* 2009;36:167–179.
9. Toohey JS. Domestic violence and rape. *Med Clin North Am.* 2008;92:1239–1252.
10. Zink T. The challenge of managing families with intimate partner violence in primary care. *Prim Care Companion J Clin Psychiatry.* 2007;9(6):410–412.
11. Bachman R, Saltzman L. Violence against women: estimates from the redesigned survey. Washington, DC: US Department of Justice; 1995.
12. Canadian Centre for Justice Statistics. Family violence in Canada: a statistical profile. Ottawa, Ontario, Canada: Statistics Canada; 2000.
13. Wheel gallery. Home of the Duluth model. Domestic Abuse and Intervention Programs Web site. http://www.theduluthmodel.org/wheelgallery.php. Accessed September 30, 2009.
14. Oriel KA, Fleming MF. Screening men for partner violence in a primary care setting. A new strategy for detecting domestic violence. *J Fam Pract.* 1998;47(3):235–236.
15. Jaffe P, Sudermann M. Child witness of women abuse: research and community responses. In: Stith S, Straus M, eds. *Understanding Partner Violence: Prevalence, Causes, Consequences, and Solutions.* Vol 3. Minneapolis, MN: National Council on Family Relations; 1995.

16. Stiles MM. Witnessing domestic violence: the effect on children. *Am Fam Physician.* 2002;66(11):2052, 2055–2056, 2058.

17. Chang JC, Buranosky R, Dado D, et al. Helping women victims of intimate partner violence: comparing the approaches of two health care settings. *Violence Victims.* 2009;24(2):193–203.

18. Gillum TL, Sun CJ, Woods AB. Can a health clinic-based intervention increase safety in abused women? Results from a pilot study. *J Womens Health.* 2009;18(8):1259–1264.

Chapter 18

Prevention of Family Violence

Judith A. Gravdal, MD
Jo Marie Reilly, MD

INTRODUCTION

Violence has an impact on individuals, families, communities, and society at large. Physicians and other healthcare workers lead the efforts to prevent family violence (FV), including: (1) identification of risk factors (both for victims and perpetrators), (2) alertness to early signs and symptoms of FV, (3) assessment for violence in families, (4) management of the sequelae of violence to minimize morbidity and mortality, (5) knowledge of referral and community resources, and (6) advocacy for societal change that can promote a violence-free environment.

Prevention requires multi-level, multidisciplinary efforts. The healthcare community must collaborate with professionals in other fields, such as public health, education, social services, law enforcement, advocacy, and politics, to accomplish the goal of violence prevention. Violence arises from historical, cultural, interpersonal and intrapersonal stresses, and belief systems. Health and socioeconomic factors impact on and are impacted by FV. The traditional medical model alone cannot address violence prevention.[1,2]

The ecological approach encompasses many of the components of prevention. This model illustrates the interplay among the individual, relationships, family, community, and society. A number of authors have discussed this concept in general terms and, more specifically, with respect to the components of FV: child abuse, intimate partner violence (IPV), and elder abuse.[3-7]

Five key components have been identified: (1) identify and modify individual risky behaviors and risk factors; (2) foster healthy relationships and healthy families; (3) make public places safe (schools, work, community/neighborhood); (4) deal with cultural/structural issues: e.g., gender, race, faith; and (5) address economic barriers to access to education, health care, and other critical needs.[3] In this chapter, an ecological model of violence prevention strategies is proposed that illustrates the interplay of violence prevention strategies across the life-cycle and highlights the interactions of family, interpersonal relationships, education, health care, community, and society (including the legal system). Figure 18–1 depicts the model.

This chapter addresses the primary, secondary, tertiary, and quaternary prevention of FV across the life-cycle. Violence intervention and prevention strategies are discussed in the context of a life-cycle ecological model (Figure 18–1) and are categorized according to those that are education based, healthcare based, community based, and society and legal based.

Violence remains one of the most significant public health issues in the United States and has received much attention, particularly over the past 4 decades. A comprehensive prevention strategy, however, has proven challenging and elusive. The literature on violence prevention is not evidence based, has many gaps, and, although it crosses many disciplines, it has rarely been interdisciplinary. A cohesive and integrated approach to violence prevention is needed but does not yet exist.

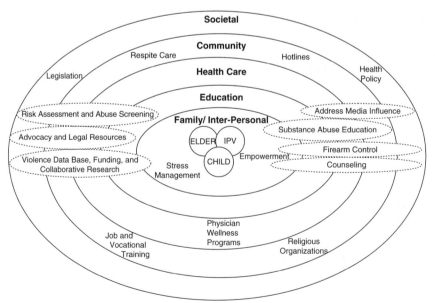

Figure 18–1 Ecologic model of violence and prevention strategies across the life-cycle.

PRIMARY PREVENTION

Primary prevention is defined as the prevention of violence before it occurs.[8] Strategies include education, skills development, and resource allocation. Increasing awareness about healthy relationships, the risk factors for violent behaviors, and alternatives to violence can promote primary prevention among individuals and caregivers within the community. Consciousness raising of what constitutes maltreatment and abuse is a crucial aspect of this level of prevention. Candib underscored both the challenge and the importance of focusing on primary prevention.[9]

Primary prevention assumes that everyone is at risk of experiencing violence and can contribute to risk reduction. *Risk factors* identify those at above-average risk, with the goal of earlier deployment of primary prevention strategies. The following general risk factors have been investigated: alcohol and/or substance abuse by either victim or perpetrator, firearms in the home, poverty, economic difficulty and/or financial dependency, mental health problems in either victim or perpetrator, history of family violence, alternative lifestyle, and exposure to violent content in media or Internet. These may apply to the victim, the perpetrator, and/or to the community.[10]

Child abuse and maltreatment risk is the "failure to act on the part of a caretaker or parent which results in death, harm or maltreatment of a child."[11] It increases when the following situations are present: low maternal education, parental psychiatric disturbances, presence of a stepfather, single-parent status, young age of mother, child with mental or physical disabilities, and large family size.[12] As the number of risk factors increases, the proportion of children abused increases.[11]

Intimate partner violence (IPV) is the abuse of power and control within intimate relationships. The perpetrator treats the victim as an object. Gender inequality results in a predominance of violence by male partners against women, but IPV also includes female violence against males and violence within same-sex relationships.[13] The following risk factors, along with the general ones, place adults at an increased risk for interpartner violence, abuse, and maltreatment: mental health problems in either victim or perpetrator, pregnancy, gender, age, history of dating violence, history of childhood sexual abuse, and sexual orientation.[13]

Elder abuse and maltreatment, the youngest field in the study of FV, was first described in 1975.[14] Elder abuse includes financial abuse, physical abuse, sexual abuse, emotional abuse, neglect, abandonment, and self neglect. Agreement on a clear definition for either clinical or research purposes remains a challenge.[15] The risk for elder abuse is increased by financial dependency (of either victim or perpetrator), educational level of caregiver, and mental health problems in either victim or perpetrator. Contextual factors, such as long-standing IPV, substance abuse, caregiver stress, and abuse by an aggressive dementia patient, for instance, have been identified.[16,17] Significant others, other family members, and paid caregivers (either in the victim's home or in the institution where the victim lives) have been identified as the relationships of highest concern.[16]

Interventions

Prevention strategies that raise awareness of abuse across the life-span fall into several categories: education based, physician/healthcare provider based, community based, and societal or legal.

Education-based violence reduction curricula have been introduced from elementary school through college. Elementary school curricula tend to inform children of their right to personal safety, personal boundaries, injury prevention, and building trusting relationships with others.[18] Early identification of at-risk children, with close monitoring for signs and symptoms of abuse and reinforcement of violence reduction strategies underscores children's right to personal safety.[19] Important violence prevention strategies in elementary school also include "bully intervention"[20] and substance abuse prevention.[21]

Teen-based pregnancy prevention programs have been shown to provide primary prevention for abuse. Educating teens (both girls and boys) on family planning methods and parenthood may decrease the likelihood of becoming a parent with limited physical, emotional, social, or financial resources to care for a child.[22]

Teaching children about safe and healthy relationships is a violence prevention strategy. As mandated reporters, teachers need training to identify risk factors, risky behaviors, and victim needs. They must know what resources are available and how to make referrals.[23] Teachers require emotional support and resources to cope with the challenges of working with families and children who are victims of violence.[23]

The PREVENT (Preventing Violence through Education, Networking and Technical assistance) program is an example of a curricular intervention for healthcare and community providers that addresses primary prevention of child abuse and IPV.[24] Educational strategies must both inform individuals of their rights and support expectations for healthy relationships.

Educational efforts to provide anticipatory guidance for elders, their family members, and their caregivers can identify the needs and wishes of elderly persons. Knowledge and skills education, along with stress management for caregivers, may prevent abuse and mistreatment.[15]

Physicians and other healthcare providers need specific training to meet their obligations to deploy prevention strategies within the loci of their clinical practices. The importance of primary prevention of violence and the risk factors that put people at risk of violence should be introduced early in their professional education. The curricula in all healthcare training should include raising awareness, exposure to victims of violence, and knowledge about resources for violence prevention.[25] Training should ensure that healthcare providers demonstrate the ability to perform appropriate and sensitive histories and physicals that assess the presence of risk factors for FV, such as a history of FV, mental illness, access to firearms, and substance abuse screening.[25] Healthcare providers' assessments should recognize physical and emotional symptoms that may suggest abuse. They must be able to dispense patient education and guidance to prevent FV.

Both the Liaison Committee on Medical Education (LCME) and Accreditation Council for Graduate Medical Education (ACGME) have statements about violence education in trainee curricula.[26,27] IPV education during family medicine and obstetrics and gynecology residency training has been associated with increased rates of screening.[28] Professional education about elder abuse occurs more frequently in family medicine residencies than in internal medicine or emergency medicine.[29] Literature that identifies and evaluates the competencies needed by healthcare providers has begun to appear.[30,31]

Specialty organizations have had varying approaches to the problem of family violence. Table 18–1 provides links to position statements by the primary medical specialties that encounter FV victims, witnesses, and perpetrators. Some child abuse and IPV prevention strategies described in the literature include (1) education during prenatal visits and prior to hospital discharge[32]; (2) home visits after hospital discharge to assist new parents in their adjustment to the responsibilities of parenthood[33]; (3) parenting classes during pregnancy and postpartum[33]; (4) maternal/paternal support groups; (5) universal screening at well child and well woman visits for risk factors[12,34]; (6) teaching caregivers/parents appropriate bathing and toilet training methods[35]; (7) legally mandated reporting of suspected child abuse and IPV[36]; (8) parental guidance about violence on or involving TV, movies, music, video games, the Internet, and various public "icons"[37–39]; (9) teaching all healthcare providers the signs, symptoms, and resources for suspected child abuse and IPV; and (10) recognition of "shaken baby syndrome."[40]

The primary prevention of elder abuse may be addressed by healthcare providers in a number of settings. These include office visits, extended-care facilities, inpatient facilities, and home visits or visits from home healthcare providers.

Community-based intervention programs are also critical to the prevention of abuse across the life cycle. Public awareness campaigns, public service announcements, advertisements, and media messages have been deployed

Table 18–1 Position Statements

Statements by professional organization and expert bodies on violence prevention provide insight into specialty perception of and commitment to preventing violence. Information about key professional society statements follows in alphabetical order.

American Academy of Family Physicians:
http://www.aafp.org/online/en/home/policy/policies/v/violencepositionpaper.html

The American Academy of Pediatrics:
http://pediatrics.aappublications.org/cgi/reprint/peds.2009-0943v1

American College of Emergency Physicians:
http://www.acep.org/practres.aspx?id=29184

The American College of Obstetrics and Gynecology:
Technical Bulletin (Number 209) was published in August 1995 and a Sexual Assault Bulletin (Number 242) was published in 1997.

A Fact Sheet on interpersonal violence against women has been published:
http://www.acop.org/departments/dept-notice.cfm?recno=17&bulletin=186

A "Violence Against Women" home page is maintained:
http://www.acog.org/departments/dept_web.cfm?recno=17.

American College of Physicians:
http://www.acponline.org/ppvl/policies/e000205.doc

The American Geriatrics Society:
http://www.americangeriatrics.org/products/positionpapers/elder_abusePF.shtml

American Medical Association:
http://www.ama-assn.org/ama/pub/physician-resources/public-health/promoting-healthy-lifestyles/violence-prevention.shtml

Centers for Disease Control and Prevention:
http://www.cdc.gov/ViolencePrevention/index.html

Surgeon General:
http://www.mentalhealth.samhsa.gov/youthviolence/orderform.asp

World Heath Organization:
http://www.who.int/violence_injury_prevention

as violence prevention strategies.[41] Community-based programs include efforts to monitor and modify media violence on TV, movies, music, the Internet, and computer games.[37,39] Parental attendance at parenting classes and involvement in community support groups from birth through elementary school years can prevent abuse.[42] Societal changes have led to the decreased availability of extended family networks to mentor and aid in child-rearing. As a result, community programs offering parenting education and family support are essential. Job training programs and incentives for young adults to finish school result in primary prevention in the following ways: less financial strain; improved self-esteem; and increased motivation for young at-risk adults. Gang intervention programs also are critical to violence prevention. One such program is "Jobs for the Future," which emphasizes jobs as a means of creating personal identity and increasing the economic security, training, and rehabilitation of at-risk or gang youth.[43] Community-based counseling and support for at-risk parents who have themselves been victims of child abuse are promising.[44]

Religious organizations often provide information about violence prevention and resources. With appropriate training, clergy and lay leaders can contribute to the prevention of family and societal violence.[45]

An awareness of and access to resources such as community-based day care and respite care options contribute to violence prevention. Social supports for the elderly and their formal and informal caregivers are critical. A model of integrating social (adult protective services), criminal justice, and medical expertise, the VAST (Vulnerable Adult Specialist Team) has been found helpful, as discussed by Mosqueda.[46] Linking home- and community-based support services to assessment for risk of abuse as described should be further studied.[47]

Societal, even global, commitment is necessary for effective FV prevention. A prerequisite to preventing FV is acknowledging and addressing the impact of structural and global violence.[48] The World Health Organization (WHO) report asserts that "preventing one type of violence can therefore help to prevent other types of violence, and by addressing the cross-cutting risk factors it is possible to help reduce all forms of violence."[49] Risk factors for societal violence have been delineated,[10] and, as with interpersonal abuse, they include cultural norms, power differentials, poverty, social isolation, substance abuse, and access to firearms.

Legal reforms and strengthening of the criminal justice system can serve as primary prevention strategies. Enhancing police knowledge and responsiveness may reduce the risk of FV. Ongoing IPV training and awareness for police and law enforcement officers will allow them to be more effective when they respond to domestic calls in the home and workplace.[50] Legislation can increase support for safety-net programs and provide funding for personnel trained to intervene in high-risk situations. Background screening, training, and surveillance of both informal and formal caregivers should be expanded and may help to prevent elder abuse.

SECONDARY PREVENTION

The definition of *secondary prevention* includes intervention with high-risk populations, in risky situations, and by prompt response to victims and perpetrators.[8] Secondary prevention highlights plans for intervention after maltreatment or abuse has been identified and requires a high index of suspicion. Ideally, assessment or screening would lead to early diagnosis, to the prevention of recurrence by interrupting the cycle of violence,[2] and to the amelioration or mitigation of harm.

Child abuse may manifest in poor school performance (either academic or emotional). Precocious behavior should alert the clinician to the possibility of abuse, as should new and sudden changes in personality or behavior.[51] IPV may present with any or a combination of the symptoms listed. Elder abuse may manifest in many ways. In addition to the common signs and symptoms, an important indicator of elder abuse that may be overlooked is self-neglect.[52-54]

Interventions

Secondary prevention relies on the ability of healthcare personnel, teachers, community members, social workers, and law enforcement officers to properly identify and refer victims and their families to appropriate resources.

Education-based interventions for secondary prevention build on the previously discussed strategies. School-based efforts are pivotal. Teachers, counselors, and administrators are charged with creating a school environment that models safety and respect, responds early and effectively to violence, and encourages reporting.[55] All individuals should be aware of the signs of FV, and schools should provide and reinforce information, including early diagnosis through screening, awareness and index of suspicion, prevention of recurrence, prevention of harm, and awareness of cultural and behavioral change that ends the cycle of violence.[56]

Physician and healthcare provider approaches to secondary prevention of child abuse include not only screening for risk factors using screening tools such as those discussed in Chapter 4 but also careful observation of behavioral and developmental variances that may suggest abuse. The requirement to report suspicion must be reinforced and emergency department personnel are required by the Joint Commission on Accreditation of Healthcare Organization (JCAHO)'s 1992 mandate to report all signs and suspicions of physical abuse in children.[36]

IPV screening for risk factors at all well-woman visits (Chapter 16) has been recommended as an office-based secondary prevention strategy. The use of IPV reading materials and resources (in safe locations, unseen by perpetrators) in physician offices, hospitals, emergency departments, and outpatient settings, such as mammography suites, also address secondary prevention. These materials should provide information about counseling, shelters, victim hotlines, and relationships with local police.

Physicians and other healthcare providers must maintain a high index of suspicion for possible elder abuse. Perpetrators also may present as patients, and healthcare personnel have a unique opportunity to explore the stressors faced by the caregivers of elderly persons, to consider the risk factors that may be present, to encourage self-care, and to advise about available assistance. Table 18–2 lists strategies for the healthcare provider.

Community-based efforts to educate the public about both the cycle of violence and the attributes of healthy relationships are important strategies

Table 18–2 Strategies for the Healthcare Provider

Office
    Active use of assessment tools
    Identify risk/history on problem list
    Patient education
    Staff education
    Locate referral options
Education
    CME
    Self-care strategies to prevent burnout
Research
    Identify opportunities to participate
Societal
    Identify local resources
    Know applicable statutes
    Lobby for resources and legislation
Web-based Resources
    www.ndvh.org
    www.rainn.org
    www.endabuse.org
    www.ncadv.org
    www.nnedv.org
    www.fvsai.org
    www.nnvawi.org
    www.inpea.net
    www.ncea.aoa.gov
    CDC Resources and Programs:
        http://origin.cdc.gov/ViolencePrevention/index.html
        http://origin.cdc.gov/ViolencePrevention/overview
ACE: Academic Centers of Excellence on Youth Violence Prevention Choose Respect
    http://www.cdc.gov/violenceprevention/ACE/goals.html
DELTA: Domestic Violence Prevention Enhancement and Leadership Through Alliances
    http://www.cdc.gov/ncipc/Delta/default.htm

in the secondary prevention of FV. Workplace harassment training may be useful. Specific to elder abuse, aid organizations and respite options are important.[57,58] State adult protective services and elder abuse hotline contact information must be widely publicized. Mandated reporting requirements and processes that pertain to child and elder abuse must become public knowledge.

Society's commitment to supporting the characteristics of a safe and equal relationship underpins secondary prevention efforts. Negotiation and fairness, nonthreatening and respectful behavior, trust and support, honesty and accountability, responsible parenting, shared responsibility, economic partnership, and a commitment to nonviolence are features of such relationships, as identified by the Domestic Abuse Intervention Program in Duluth, MN.[59] Awareness of, and intervention to alter, power and control tactics, such as the use of threats, economic control, manipulation, isolation, undermining, or destruction of self-confidence, dominance, and attribution of blame, can decrease violence. Interventions to prevent societal violence are usually nonclinical, but healthcare workers must be engaged in this work. The influence of role modeling (intentional and unintentional) in the political arena, popular media (such as music, film, and television), and sports and other personality "icons" requires research and consideration.[55] Newer media, such as the Internet, online social networking, texting, and Twittering deserve investigation.

Secondary interventions relate strongly to the legal sector. Legal reform and continued training for law enforcement personal and other appropriate public servants are ongoing efforts. The recent special reports of the National Institute of Justice highlight efforts in this field.[60,61] Society must continue to advocate and uphold laws that protect every individual's rights, particularly those who are dependent (e.g., children and the elderly) and those who typically have not enjoyed equal rights (women, minorities, and other marginalized populations). Victims need education and assistance in obtaining restraining orders (Chapter 21). Jurisdictions must ensure that orders are served in a timely and appropriate fashion. Tactics must be developed to strengthen and support the integrity of the victim's court testimony. Laws to protect people both at home and in the workplace are needed. The option of allowing and encouraging the police to file a complaint and provide court testimony are important secondary prevention strategies.

TERTIARY PREVENTION

The definition of tertiary prevention encompasses the consequences of violence, the amelioration of sequelae, and the prevention of both further victimization and transformation of victims into perpetrators. Tertiary prevention is actually intervention after the fact.[8] At this stage, violence has occurred, recurred, and has, in effect, become a chronic problem. The goals are to: (1) prevent or ameliorate the sequelae of violence, (2) prevent further damage/complications, (3) limit both physical and social consequences, and (4) understand and manage violence as a chronic disease.

Interventions

Education-based interventions for tertiary prevention build on the previously discussed strategies. Advocacy, educational efforts, and programs that provide support and care for victims fit into this area.

The establishment of safe and healthy living and learning environments for children should permit them to do well in non-violent environments. Shelters and homes for women and children must be identified and supported. State child protective services require adequate funding and oversight so that children can be placed and monitored in safe living communities.[62]

Ideally, efforts to heal, rehabilitate, and empower victims of IPV decrease the risk of future violence. Vocational and job training programs help to provide financial independence and stability. Shelters and safe living environments for women and their children should help lead to self-sufficiency.[63,64]

Educating the caregivers of the elderly is critical to both identifying and intervening in violence in this population. Since the prevalence of abuse among vulnerable elders is high, family members, caregivers, and community members must consider the possibility of abuse.[65-68] Assessing the patient or situation can lead to physician intervention and reporting to appropriate agencies. Agencies and organizations have additional resources to prevent further injury and harm.

A comprehensive discussion of tertiary prevention requires consideration of the perpetrators. Identifying perpetrators and addressing their psychological needs is important. Bell and Orcutt summarized the evidence for a link between posttraumatic stress disorder (PTSD) and the perpetration of IPV by men.[69] Efforts to rehabilitate perpetrators include perpetrator education, vocational training, counseling, and anger management courses. These strategies have shown mixed results.

Healthcare providers can send a strong message to victims, perpetrators, and the community. Intrinsic to the tertiary prevention of FV is the healthcare provider's commitment to prevent the sequelae of violence and the physical and social consequences of violence. Advocacy skills can and should be taught at all levels of professional education. Physicians and other healthcare providers are respected community leaders, and their role carries a special responsibility to act and advocate for violence prevention through activities such as community talks, media presentations, writing letters to the editor or health columns, serving as key contacts for local, state, and federal politicians, and serving as leaders within their specialty organizations.

Community-based tertiary interventions include those identified in the section on secondary prevention.

Societal commitment to effective tertiary prevention requires, at a minimum, the following: (1) surveillance systems that track fatal and nonfatal injuries and their causes, (2) "guidelines for conducting community surveys on injury and violence,"[49] and (3) educational system initiatives for the prevention of violence in schools.

Legal strategies, such as victim assistance programs, can contribute to tertiary prevention. One example of a program that assists families dealing with FV is the Illinois Victim's Economic Security & Safety Act (VESSA).[70] An employee may request a VESSA leave that provides excused time away from work for up to 12 weeks if an employee or employee's family member is a victim of domestic or sexual violence (provided the employee is not the perpetrator).

QUATERNARY PREVENTION

Quaternary prevention is the prevention of iatrogenic harm to individuals, communities, and healthcare providers.[71,72] The first aspect of quaternary prevention addresses the avoidance of harm to victims by a healthcare professional. One example of such prevention is education in knowledge, skills, and attitudes that enable healthcare professionals to avoid revictimizing individuals through an inappropriate verbal or nonverbal approach, by the lack of knowledge, or through a misguided attitude. Quaternary prevention, which may be an unfamiliar concept to many, restates the commitment of healthcare workers to the fundamental tenet of medicine, *Primum non nocere* ("First do no harm").[73]

The second aspect of quaternary prevention is equipping the provider to cope with the stress of dealing with victims of violence. Violence intervention and prevention work is challenging for physicians and other healthcare providers, particularly with respect to the management of their own emotional response and sometimes their own past personal experiences, their competency, and their time. Healthcare workers, including medical students, may find themselves professionally helping victims while personally dealing with FV. Prevention of and early intervention for both burnout and "compassion fatigue" are important.[74]

The concern about inadvertently harming vulnerable victims in the process of attempting to provide them with medical care has been raised to some degree in the IPV literature.[73] How healthcare providers can affect a victim's feelings, actions, and future safety is of concern. Another challenge is how appropriate reporting of abuse may affect someone's future safety. Many women are afraid to report their victimization for fear of retribution. Not all healthcare providers are sensitive to this concern or to the physical and emotional damage that IPV victims face. Further studies and education are needed in this area.

Healthcare providers' needs also must be considered. Physicians identify negative feelings in response to caring for victims of IPV.[75] These negative feelings combined with inadequate (or no) training and a possible personal history of child abuse, IPV, or other exposure to violence likely will affect the healthcare provider's ability to address the patient's needs. "Compassion fatigue" may alter the provider's ability to recognize and report FV.[74] Healthcare providers who experience burnout, stress, and/or frequent trauma, death, or patient victimization in their work may be at increased risk for such burnout. Training in the signs and symptoms of burnout, physician wellness programs, and early recognition of the effect on healthcare providers is critical to quaternary violence prevention.[76]

CHALLENGES AND GAPS

The literature on violence prevention is not evidence based, has many gaps, and is multidisciplinary but rarely interdisciplinary. Healthcare leadership and provider education need to address these gaps. Research is needed to guide prevention strategies.

Provider Education

Medical schools are accredited by the Liaison Commission on Medical Education (LCME), which states in section ED-20 that the medical school "curriculum must prepare students for their role in addressing the medical consequences of common societal problems, for example, providing instruction in the diagnosis, prevention, appropriate reporting, and treatment of violence and abuse."[26] Little is known about how this requirement is accomplished and how educational initiatives at the medical school level have been evaluated. Graduate (residency) medical education is accredited by the Accreditation Council for Graduate Medical Education (ACGME).[27] The institutional requirements do not address violence education and prevention. Each specialty's program requirements address this uniquely and usually nonspecifically.

The literature about requirements for the education of other healthcare providers in violence and violence prevention is sparse. The education of community service providers, such as social workers, police, teachers, and judges, appears to be local and not standardized. Efforts to develop, test, disseminate, and evaluate curricula on the prevalence and prevention of FV is essential to violence awareness and prevention efforts.

Research

FV is an major public health concern in the United States yet most research is disease based. Investigating preventive and educational services has not received high priority. Public services and health policy are driven by evidence-based research, and gaps in violence prevention research challenge the establishment of a unified strategy for violence prevention.

The US Preventive Services Task Force (USPSTF) gives a rating of "insufficient evidence" to screening for domestic violence[77] (Chapter 16). The basis for this recommendation is that there is no good research to substantiate the benefits, assess the cost-benefit ratio, and determine the lack of harm of such screening efforts. The significant impact of violence on the quality of life, the quantity of life, and long-term sequelae has been well documented and is not contested, but most publications in the area of FV are not evidence-based, well-designed research studies. The case for cost, morbidity, and mortality reduction through early intervention and treatment seems logical but has not been made. It is not known whether early intervention is more effective than no intervention or later intervention.

Erlingsson found little variety or range in the type of scholarly investigation in understanding and preventing elder abuse.[78] The need for valid and reliable measures has been identified.[52,79] Other problems identified include lack of criteria for study populations, lack of comparison groups, lack of methodologic consistency, lack of prospective studies, and lack of outcome criteria that demonstrate the impact of interventions.[10] Pillemer and colleagues have identified many methodological issues confronting those who embark on violence research.[80] These include problems with the data sources and the nature of the available data. Meaningful research requires clear definitions, valid and reliable instruments, and appropriate and feasible outcome measures.

We do not have much in the way of outcome data that measure the success or failure of IPV prevention strategies. Research supports attitudinal shifts (e.g., a decrease in violent attitudes after educational strategies),[81,82] but it is not clear that these educational interventions decrease abusive behavior.

Collaborative, interdisciplinary research across the life-span is required. Medical and public health research must become aligned to further violence prevention initiatives.[83] Difficulty in securing reliable sources of funding at the local, state, and national levels poses a significant challenge to accumulating an evidence-based, comprehensive body of literature on FV. Long-term and longitudinal studies are needed to identify effective prevention, assessment, and treatment approaches. Research exploring opportunities to identify, intervene, and understand strategies that reduce recidivism of perpetrators is sparse. A lack of federal coordination of violence reporting and service delivery compounds the problems of abuse definitions, assessment tool identification, and outcome studies.[84]

Perhaps the gaps and needs for FV prevention are best summarized in the World Report on Violence and Health, which emphasized that violence prevention "requires political and financial commitment and may require a great deal of courage and fortitude as the many faces of violence go deep into the roots of families, societies and cultures."[48] Our efforts must be grounded in evidence-based research and further educational strategies.

REFERENCES

1. Mercy JA, Saul J. Creating a healthier future through early interventions for children. *JAMA.* 2009;301(21):2262-2264.
2. Rosenberg ML, Fenley MA, Johnson D, Short L. Bridging prevention and practice: public health and family violence. *Acad Med.* 1997;72(1 Suppl):S13-18.
3. Department of Health and Human Services. Definition of the social ecological model. Washington, DC: Centers for Disease Control and Prevention; National Center for Injury Prevention and Control Division of Violence Prevention; August 2008.
4. Little L, Kantor G. Using ecological theory to understand IPV and child maltreatment. *J Community Health Nurs.* 2002;19(3):133-145.
5. Doty MM, Meuer LN, Nguyen AL, et al. Elder abuse risk and profile of reported cases in Milwaukee County. Family Medicine Digital Resources Library Web site. http://www.fmdrl.org/index.cfm.event=c.beginBrowseD&clearSelections =1&criteria=doty#2350. Accessed November 11, 2009.
6. Heise LL. Violence against women: an integrated ecologic framework. *Violence Against Women.* 1998;4:262-290.
7. Tolan P, Gorman-Smith D, Henry D. Family violence. *Ann Rev Psychol.* 2006;57: 557-583.
8. Centers for Disease Control and Prevention Web site. http://wonder.cdc.gov/ wonder/prevguid/p0000177/p0000177.asp. Accessed November 15, 2009.
9. Candib LM. Primary violence prevention: taking a deeper look. *J Fam Pract.* 2000;49:904-906.
10. Dahlberg LL, Krug EG. Violence: a global public health problem. In Krug E, Dahlberg LL, Mercy JA, Zwi AB, Lozano R, eds. *World Report on Violence and Health.* Geneva, Switzerland: World Health Organization; 2002:1-21.
11. Child Abuse Prevention and Treatment Act Amendments (CAPTA) of 1996. PL No. 104-235.
12. Brown J, Cohen P, Johnson J. A longitudinal analysis of risk factors of child maltreatment; findings of a 17-year prospective study of officially recorded and self-reported child abuse and neglect. *Child Abuse Negl.* 1998;22:1065-1078.
13. IPV prevention and scientific info: risk and protective factors. Centers for Disease Control and Prevention Web site. http://www.cdc.gov/ncipc/dvp/ipv/ipv-risk_protective.htm. Accessed November 9, 2009.
14. Burston GR. Granny-battering. *BMJ.* 1975;3:592.
15. Nerenberg L. *Elder Abuse Prevention: Emerging Trends and Promising Strategies.* New York, NY: Springer; 2008.
16. Lachs MS, Pillmer K. Elder abuse. *Lancet.* 2004;364:1263-1272.
17. Walling AD. Intervention and treatment strategies of elder abuse. American Academy of Family Physicians Web site. http://www.aafp.org/afp/20050901/tips/ 21.html. Accessed July 7, 2009.

18. Sudermann M, Jaffee P. ASAP: a school based anti-violence prevention program. Centre for Children and Families in the Justice System Web site. http://www.lfcc.on.ca/asap.htm. Accessed November 16, 2009.

19. APA Online. APA Public Affairs Office. Two successful violence prevention programs highlight the importance of early intervention. March 9, 2003.

20. Olweus D, Limber S, Mihalic S. *Blueprints for Violence Prevention: Bullying Prevention Program.* Boulder, CO: Center for Study and Prevention of Violence; 1999.

21. National Institute on Drug Abuse. *Preventing Drug Use Among Children & Adolescents. A Research Based Guide for Parents, Educators & Community Leaders.* Washington, DC: US Department of Health and Human Services; 2003.

22. Porter A. Reducing teenage and unintended pregnancies through client-centered and family-focused school-based family planning programs. *J Pediatr Nurs.* 1998; 13(3):158–163.

23. Renk K, Liljequist L, Steinberg A, Bosco G, Phares V. Prevention of child abuse: are we doing enough? *Trauma Violence Abuse.* 2002;3;68–84.

24. Runyan CW. PREVENT: a program of the National Training Initiative on Injury and Violence Prevention. *Am J Prev Med.* 2005;29(5 Suppl 2):252–258.

25. Cohn F, Salmon M, Stobo J. *Confronting Chronic Neglect: The Education and Training of Health Professionals on Family Violence.* Washington DC: National Academies Press; 2002.

26. Teaching standards on violence and abuse. Liaison Commission on Medical Education Web site. http://www.lcme.org. Accessed November 9, 2009.

27. Emergency procedures and abuse and neglect of children. Accreditation Council for Graduate Medical Education (ACGME) Web site. http://www.acgme.org. Accessed November 9, 2009.

28. Sitterding HA, Adera T, Shields-Fobbs E. Spouse/partner violence education as a predictor of screening practices among physicians. *J Contin Educ Health Prof.* 2003;23:54–63.

29. Wagenaar DB, Rosenbaum R, Herman S, Page C. Elder abuse education in primary care residency programs: a cluster group analysis. *Fam Med.* 2009;41(7):481–486.

30. Runyan CW, Stidham SS. Core competencies for injury and violence prevention. *Injury Prev.* 2009;15:141.

31. Songer T, Stephens-Stidham S, Peek-Asa C, et al. Core competencies for injury and violence prevention. *Am J Public Health.* 2009;99(4):600–606.

32. Wallach VA. Home-based family support services: part of a comprehensive national plan to improve the overall health and safety of children. *Hawaii Med J.* 1994;53:252–253, 261.

33. Dubowitz H, King H. Family violence. a child centered, family-focused approach. *Pediatr Clin North Am.* 1995;42(1):153–166.

34. Thompson RS, Rivera FP, Thompson DC, et al. Identification and management of domestic violence: a randomized trial. *Am J Prev Med.* 2000;19(4):253–262.

35. Reisinger KS, Bires JA. Anticipatory guidance in pediatric practice. *Pediatrics.* 1980;66:889–892.

36. Joint Commission on Accreditation of Healthcare Organizations. *Accreditation Manual for Hospitals.* Oakbrook Terrace, IL: Joint Commission on Accreditation of Healthcare Organizations; 1992. *Standards;* vol 1.

37. National Association for the Education of Young Children. *Position Statement. Media Violence in Children's Lives.* Washington, DC: National Association for the Education of Young Children; 1994.

38. Kaiser Family Foundation. Children get a mixed message from athletes, both on and off the field [media release]; October 12, 2000.

39. Anderson A, Carnagey N. Exposure to violent media: the effects of songs with violent lyrics on aggressive thoughts and feelings. *J Pers Soc Disord.* 2003;960-971.

40. Newton A, Vandeen A. Update on child maltreatment: shaken baby syndrome. *Curr Opin Pediatr.* 2005;17:246-251.

41. Thomas E. Beyond blame: media literacy as violence prevention. Center for Media Literacy Web site. http://www.medialit.org/reading_roomarticle93.html. Accessed November 16, 2009.

42. Prevent Child Abuse America Web site. An approach. http://www.preventchild-abuse.org. Accessed November 6, 2009.

43. Jobs not jails. Homeboy Industries Web site. http://www.homeboy-industries.org. Accessed November 9, 2009.

44. Vuong L, Silva F, Marchionna S. Focus: views from the National Council on Crime and Delinquency. Children Exposed to Violence. August 2009. Available at http://www.safestartcenter.org/resources/. Accessed October 8, 2010.

45. Virtus training. The National Catholic Risk Retention Group Web site. http://www.scdiocese.org/Dioceseinfo/safeenvironment/virtustraining. Accessed November 8, 2009.

46. Mosqueda L. Advancing the field of elder mistreatment: a new model for integration of social and medical services. *Gerontologist.* 2004;44(5):703-708.

47. Shugarman LR, Fries BE, Wolf RS, Morris JN. Identifying older people at risk of abuse during routine screening practices. *J Am Geriatr Soc.* 2003;51(1): 24-31.

48. Sethi D, Marais S, Seedat M, et al. *Handbook for the Documentation of Interpersonal Violence Prevention Programmes.* Geneva, Switzerland: Department of Injuries and Violence Prevention, World Health Organization; 2004.

49. Bartolomeos K. *Third Milestones of a Global Campaign for Violence Prevention Report.* Geneva, Switzerland: World Health Organization; 2007.

50. Evaluation of law enforcement and prosecution programs, Violence Against Women Act (STOP grants). Institute for Law and Justice Web site. http://www.ilj.org/focus_areas/violent_crime.html. Accessed November 8, 2009.

51. Dominguez R, Nelke C, Perry B. *Encyclopedia of Crime and Punishment: Sexual Abuse of Children.* Vol 1. Sage Publications; 2001.

52. Dyer CB, Pickens S, Burnett J. Vulnerable elders: when it is no longer safe to live alone. *JAMA.* 2007;298(12):1448-1450.

53. Gill TM. Elder self-neglect: medical emergency or marker of extreme vulnerability? *JAMA.* 2009;302(5):570-571.

54. Dong XQ, Simon M, deLeon CM, et al. Elder self-neglect and abuse and mortality risk in a community-dwelling population. *JAMA.* 2009;302(5):517-526.

55. DeJong W. *Preventing Interpersonal Violence Among Youth: An Introduction to School, Community and Mass Media Strategies.* Washington, DC: National Institute of Justice, US Department of Justice; 1994.

56. CAPS: Child Abuse Prevention Services Training Programs Web site. http://www.capsli.org/prevention.php. Accessed November 16, 2009.

57. Dyer CB, Heisler CJ, Hill CA, Kim LC. Community approaches to elder abuse. *Clin Geriatr Med.* 2005;429–447.

58. Richard L, Gauvin L, Gosselin C, et al. Integrating the ecological approach in hearth promotion for older adults: a survey of programs aimed at elder abuse prevention, falls prevention, and appropriate medication use. *Int J Public Health.* 2008;53(1):46–56.

59. Domestic Abuse Intervention Programs Web site. http://www.theduluthmodel.org/wheelgallery.php. Accessed November 15, 2009.

60. *Legal Interventions in Family Violence: Research Finds and Policy Implications.* National Institute of Justice Web site. Available at http://ncjrs.gov/pdffiles/171666.pdf. Accessed October 18, 2009.

61. Klein AR. Practical implications of current domestic violence research for law enforcement, prosecutors and judges. National Institute of Justice Web site. http://www.ncjrs.gov/pdffiles1/nij/223572.pdf. Accessed October 18, 2009.

62. Child Abuse Victimization: OVC Help Series. National Center for Victims of Crime Web site. http://www.ojp.usdoj.gov.ovc/publications. Accessed November 16, 2009.

63. American Medical Association. *Diagnostic and Treatment Guidelines on Domestic Violence.* 1–12. 2002. Available at http://archfami.ama-assn.org/cgi/reprint/1/1/39. Accessed October 8, 2010.

64. Wolfe DA, Jaffe PG. Emerging strategies in the prevention of domestic violence. *Future Child.* 1999;9(3):133–144.

65. O'Malley TA, Everitt DE, O'Malley HC, Campion EW. Identifying and preventing family-mediated abuse and neglect of elderly persons. *Ann Intern Med.* 1983;98:988–1005.

66. Wolf RS. Elder abuse: ten years later. *J Am Geriatr Soc.* 1988;36(8):758–762.

67. Donohue W, Dibble J, Schiamberg L. A social capital approach to the prevention of elder mistreatment. *J Elder Abuse Negl.* 2008;20(1):1–23.

68. Cooper C, Manela M, Katona C, Livingston G. Screening for elder abuse in dementia in the LASER-AD study: prevalence, correlates and validation of instruments. *Int J Geriatr Psychiatry.* 2008;23:283–288.

69. Bell KM, Orcutt HK. Posttraumatic stress disorder and male-perpetrated intimate partner violence. *JAMA.* 2009;302(5):562–564.

70. Illinois Department of Labor Web site. http://www.state.il.us/agency/idol/forms/PDFS/vessaout.pdf. Accessed November 15, 2009.

71. Jamoulle M. Quaternary prevention. Available at http://www.ulb.ac.be/esp/mfsp/quat-en. htm. Accessed November 15, 2009.

72. Santiago LM. Quaternary prevention. European Union of General Practitioners/Family Physicians Web site. 2008. Available at http://www.uemo.org/members/docs/2008/08-040/ 2008-040.doc. Accessed November 15, 2009.

73. Kilo CM, Larson EB. Exploring the harmful effects of health care. *JAMA.* 2009;302(1):89–91.

74. Pfifferling JH, Gilley K. Overcoming compassion fatigue. *Fam Pract Manage.* 2000;7:39–46.

75. Garimella RN, Plichta SB, Houseman C, Garzon L. How physicians feel about assisting female victims of intimate-partner violence. *Acad Med.* 2002;77(12 Pt 1): 1262–1265.

76. Spickard A, Gabbe S, Christensen J. Mid career burnout in generalist and specialist physicians. *JAMA.* 2002;288:1447–1450.

77. Nelson HD, Nygren P, McInerney Y, Klein J. Screening women and elderly adults for family and intimate partner violence: A review of the evidence for the US Preventive Services Task Force. *Ann Intern Med.* 2004;140(5):387–396.

78. Erlingsson C. Searching for elder abuse: a systematic review of database citations. *J Elder Abuse Negl.* 2007;19(3–4):59–78.

79. Cooper C, Selwood A, Livingston G. The prevalence of elder abuse and neglect: a systematic review. *Age Ageing.* 2008;37:151–160.

80. Pillemer KA, Mueller-Johnson KU, Mock SE, et al. Interventions to Prevent Elder Mistreatment. In: Doll LS, Bonzo SE, Sleet DA, Mercy JA, eds. *Handbook of Injury and Violence Prevention.* Secaucus, NJ: Springer; 2007:241–254.

81. Bretenbecher K. Sexual assault on college campuses: is an ounce of prevention enough? *Appl Prevent Psychol.* 2000;9:23–52.

82. Foubert JD. Longitudinal effects of rape and prevention programs on fraternity men towards behavioral intentions and behavior. *J Am College Health.* 2000;48: 158–163.

83. Lurie N, Femont A. Building bridges between medical care and public health. *JAMA.* 2009;302(1):84–86.

Chapter 19

Identification of Violence in Dental Patients

Darlene D. West, DDS
Karen M. Yoder, PhD

INTRODUCTION

The dental profession in the United States promotes routine visits every 6 or 12 months. In 2008, 71% of US residents reported seeing a dentist within the past year.[1] It is likely, therefore, that because of the frequency with which US residents visit a dentist, those who are victims of various form of family violence (FV) may continue with their regular dental visits despite exhibiting evidence of violence. Detection of such evidence during routine dental visits, therefore, should lead to intervention. Visits to a dentist or oral surgeon as a result of intimate partner violence (IPV), however, are influenced by the frequency of injuries that involve bones of the mandible or maxilla, teeth, and/or soft tissues of the mouth.[2] Nationally, 9.2% of women who have been physically abused and 16.7% of those who were raped sought care from a dentist for the injuries they sustained.[3] There are varying reports of the prevalence of head and neck injuries related to IPV. It has been reported that 68% of women who are injured by their partners had head and/or neck injuries that included fractures, bruising, and lacerations.[4] Other research documented that 94% of IPV victims sustained head and/or neck injuries.[5] Two hundred and ten women injured by IPV reported the following types of injury, some reporting more than one type: lip (29%), face (21%), neck (14%), tongue (5%), broken teeth (15%), broken jaw (7%), lost teeth (5%), and other injuries, including dislocated jaw, black eye, and broken nose (3%).[6]

Based on these data, it is likely that dentists will encounter victims of FV—children, partners, elders, developmentally disabled individuals, and other vulnerable family members—in their practices. According to the American Dental Association (ADA) Principles of Ethics and Code of Professional Conduct, dentists are obliged to become familiar with the signs of abuse and neglect, including IPV, and to report suspected cases to the proper authorities, as required by state law.[7] The American Dental Education Association has a policy statement encouraging dental educators to teach about child abuse/neglect and IPV, including familiarity with signs and symptoms, and to provide information on state and federal regulations.[8] However, there has been little research concerning documentation of dentists' ability and willingness to effectively identify and intervene when violence is suspected. In a random national sample of 321 dentists, 47% reported suspecting one or more patients had been a victim of FV, and 19% said that even when the patient(s) had signs of trauma s/he did not initiate any conversation to screen for FV.[9] Dentists reported that the primary deterrents to pursuing the subject of FV were that the patient was accompanied by a partner or children (77%), the dentist felt s/he lacked training in identifying IPV (68%), and the dentist was concerned about offending the patient (66%).[9]

VICTIMS' EXPECTATIONS OF THE DENTAL PROFESSION

Small studies indicate that victims of IPV want dentists to be alert to their plight and to initiate a conversation about their injuries. One hundred and twelve victims of abuse who were residing in 15 shelters in northern Texas responded to a questionnaire.[6] Seventy-six percent had injuries in the head and neck area, and more than half of them had seen a dentist while their injuries were visible. However, 89% were not asked about their injuries. Sixty-nine percent said that they preferred to be asked about their injuries and reported that they wanted the abuse to be recognized and wanted to receive assistance or referral for help. Those who saw a dentist for their injuries were asked if they had a preference as to the gender of a dentist they might see in the future for an injury. Most had no preference (75%), 16.5% preferred a male dentist, and 8.5% preferred a woman.[6]

It is important for the dental team to be aware of the long-term effects of childhood sexual abuse to help make patients' dental visits more tolerable. Survivors of childhood sexual abuse report frequent cancellations of dental appointments because of anxiety. Anxiety related to dental treatment may be the result of the parallels between the abusive situation and the process of receiving dental care: the patient lies passively in a chair with someone working above him or her in close proximity, and the mouth is intruded upon. Dental providers can help patients adapt to the situation by asking questions that will assist them in articulating their discomfort, such as "Are you comfortable?" or "Is there anything that you need?"[10]

DENTISTS' ROLE IN GATHERING EVIDENCE, DOCUMENTATION, AND TESTIFYING

In the context of recent enhanced interest in forensic dentistry in the dental community, perhaps as a result of the role some dentists have played in forensic identification of victims of mass disasters, more dentists seem to be aware of other dental injuries, including those inflicted in IPV. Dental professionals are likely to observe the aftermath of this underreported, widespread offense in their daily practice because "the majority of injuries, found in the head and neck area, are clearly visible to the dentist."[11] The problem, as stated previously, is a lack of training in identifying IPV (68%). Recognition is the key to identification. It requires awareness of the problem and of the signs and symptoms of IPV, followed by an understanding of the recording, reporting, and referral processes before management and treatment can be started.

Patient Profile

The *2007 National Coalition Against Domestic Violence* report states that approximately 85% of IPV victims are females, most often victimized by someone they know.[12] Furthermore, of the 1.3 million women who will experience physical assault by an intimate partner, women who are 19 to 29 years of age are at the greatest risk of nonfatal IPV.[12,13] However, only about a quarter of all physical assaults perpetrated against females by intimate partners are reported to the police.[12] This underreporting could be reduced by the intervention of the dental community. The dental professional who is willing to recognize the possibility of IPV when interviewing the individual patient who presents with injuries suggesting IPV, and then documents the findings, can make a difference. Dentists should be especially diligent when the patient fits the identified profile. However, FV can affect anyone, not just those in the demographic group just described. The physical injuries associated with FV can be seen in children of all ages as well as older adults, including the disabled and the infirm. IPV also is seen in males and should be recognized; however, women are described as being at greater risk for nonaccidental trauma, and, in fact, "the battered woman syndrome" has been described as a result of the prevalence of females who sustain recurrent physical abuse at the hands of their male partners.[14] Nonetheless, dentists should routinely screen all patients for FV who present with soft or hard tissue injuries in and around the face and neck and the oral cavity, including children and adults, males and females.[15] Whether in the hospital emergency department or in a private practice, the involvement of the dentist is essential.

Description of Injuries

Multiple studies confirm that, although the diagnosis of IPV is difficult because there are no "clearly defined signs and symptoms," there is a "statistically significant association between head, neck, and facial (HNF) injuries and DV."[3,4,10] The HNF injuries from nonaccidental intentional trauma have been reported in multiple studies. Ranging from mild to severe, these injuries are described as follows:

- Lacerations and contusions of the head or face (the most common of all injury patterns)
- Hair loss caused by forceful pulling by a perpetrator
- Lip trauma: swelling or bruising with widespread ecchymoses of the underlying mucosal surface and torn labial or lingual frenum
- Bruising of facial tissues or edentulous ridges
- Fractured, avulsed, or subluxed teeth
- Semicircular wounds with bruising characteristic of bite-marks
- Fractures of the nasal bones
- Dislocation or fractures of the mandible or maxilla; trauma-induced malocclusion
- Injuries to the zygomaticomaxillary complex
- Black eyes, eye injuries, orbital fractures[10,14,16]

A 5-year retrospective review of 236 emergency department admissions revealed that 81% of IPV victims sustained maxillofacial injuries. The middle third of the face was the most frequent target (69%), with soft tissue injuries making up the most common type (61%). The average number of mandibular fractures per patient was 1.32, with fractures on the left side of the face more common because of the predominance of right-handed perpetrators.[17]

Additionally, there can be trauma sites in various stages of healing (i.e., scarring of the lips, bilateral bruising, radiographic evidence of fractured roots, and healed or healing facial bone or jaw fractures). Often the explanation of the trauma, whether reported by the patient or by a parent, caregiver, or spouse, will be inconsistent with the actual injury. The dentist also may observe injuries on the hands, forearms, and legs, unless the individual is wearing clothing that covers these areas. Clothing that is inconsistent with the season can be an indication that the presumed victim is covering up evidence of IPV.[17]

The dental manifestations of abuse vary according to the age, gender, and other characteristics of the victim. For example, elder abuse may manifest as broken dentures, facial irritation due to tape over lips, hand print on the face, abundant plaque and food debris in the mouth, or, in the case of sexual abuse, petechiae, palatal bruising, or torn labial frenum.[18] In children there may be signs of abuse, such as tearing of the labial frenum when a bottle is violently shoved into the mouth, which, of course, is not usually seen in adult abuse. Dental neglect has been considered a form of child abuse when there is evidence of untreated, previously diagnosed dental caries or rampant caries with multiple abscesses. The signs of sexual abuse may be similar (e.g., palatal petechiae and bruising) to that of the elderly victim. Probably of greatest concern is the violence toward those with mental and physical disabilities, who are abused and neglected at four times the rate of the general population and who have a higher incidence of oral health problems.[17]

Bite-Mark Injuries

Dentists have a unique role in the recognition, documentation, and interpretation of the bite-mark injury related to IPV. Teeth have long been used as weapons, both offensive and defensive, and the identification of the impression made by the human dentition in human skin is of great significance in the forensic sciences because it may be a link between victim and the perpetrator. The American Society of Forensic Odontology has developed recommendations to follow when recovering and preserving evidence related to bite-marks found on victims of violent crimes. Because accurate analysis of bite-mark evidence is challenging, advanced courses in forensic odontology are indicated for dentists who participate in this endeavor. Since living human skin changes rapidly because of the body's immediate responses to injury, recognizing and documenting bite-marks can be difficult. As a result of this repair process, evidence is rapidly lost; therefore, it is of paramount importance that the bite-mark evidence be collected as soon as it is identified.

Human bite-marks may vary in location, appearance, and severity. However, the dentist should follow a few basic principles when examining these patterned injuries. The bite-mark injury will resemble the form of the dental arches, having an oval or circular pattern. Upon examination, the dentist should be able to identify indentations, contusions, or lacerations made by specific teeth. These identification marks will most often appear as a double-arched pattern or uniform bruise that exhibits markings from the six upper and the six lower front teeth. With a comparison of tooth size and shape, along with shape and width of the dental arch pattern, the dentist can determine whether a bite-mark is from an adult or a child. Individual characteristics of teeth, such as missing or broken teeth, will produce bite-marks with more precise patterns that may help a dentist identify or rule out a specific individual as the perpetrator.[19]

A bite that produces an identifiable mark will begin to discolor, or bruise, as with any contusion produced by blunt force trauma. With time, the bruise will begin to change color and eventually fade. Although subject to interpretation, an attempt at using this change in observable coloration, as a way to stage or age bruises, has been cited as evidence of "continual abuse" in a court of law. This has been declared an invalid method because there are so many variables that affect the healing process, not the least of which is the severity of the injury, or, in the case of bite-marks, the force of the bite.[20]

Documentation and Reporting

Thorough documentation is vital before reporting a case of IPV. Documentation is evidence and is admissible in court. In dentistry, as in medicine, this begins with a straightforward interview of the victim. The interview is conducted in a nonthreatening private room with another sympathetic professional present (and in the absence of all family members or friends). Confidentiality is a must. Notes are recorded in the victim's own words as much as possible. In addition, notes should describe the patient's demeanor and not record "conclusions" or diagnoses such as "battered woman." Specific questions directed to the patient regarding physical violence, inflicted injuries, and safety concerns can elicit information that might not otherwise be volunteered. Names, dates, and times should be recorded and the patient's safety secured as much as possible.

Documentation also includes examination of the head and neck and other visible areas, such as hands, arms, and legs. The location, size, duration, color, and shape of the injuries are described both verbally in a written record and recorded visually with a diagram. Photographic documentation is preferable when consent is obtained, as well as relevant radiographs. Statements made by the patient that cannot be supported by the physical examination may be a red flag that the patient is a victim of IPV.

The dentist is obligated to report child abuse or elder abuse in states that have mandatory reporting laws. However, few states have such laws for IPV because of the fear that the victim will be injured more severely if the perpetrator finds out that s/he has told someone. Each state has law enforcement personnel dedicated to the investigation of FV and the prosecution of the individuals responsible.[15]

Management and Treatment Considerations

The term *family violence* encompasses abuses—assault and other coercive behaviors (see Chapters 1, 4, and 6)—directed toward any family member or other resident in the home. The prevalence of childhood sexual abuse (CSA) is estimated to be up to 13% of females and 5–10% of males. The implication for the dentist in practice is that there will be adults seeking treatment who have survived sexual abuse as children. As a result of the similarities between the abuse experience and elements of dental care—being alone in a room with the dentist, positioning in a reclined dental chair, parts of the body being touched or intruded upon, the loss of control, fear of being reprimanded—it has become necessary to outline specific strategies to make dental treatment less threatening for the survivor.[10,21]

Not all dentists are inclined or able to work with patients who are survivors of CSA, because treatment may require more time than is typically scheduled in a highly structured dental practice. As a result of the anxiety caused by dental procedures, survivors may have an increased tendency to cancel appointments. However, for the dentist who wants to help survivors overcome their fears, a number of strategies have been designed to make dental treatment more acceptable to both the dentist and the survivor:

- Establish rapport: Be sensitive to body language and nonverbal signs of anxiety
- Share control and involve the patient in treatment decisions, provide breaks in the exam and feedback, and use an agreed on "stop" signal when the patient needs to stop the exam
- Use a semi-reclined chair position allowing one foot on the floor, cover the patient with a blanket, and/or provide a mirror so that the patient can watch treatment
- Avoid latex gloves (that smell like condoms) and use another material; avoid use of aftershave or perfume
- Allow a person or friend in the room during treatment (as long as the person is not the abuser)[10,21]

DENTAL PROGRAMS AND ORGANIZATIONS FOR EDUCATION, SUPPORT, AND CONSULTATION

Prevent Abuse Through Dental Awareness

Prevent Abuse and Neglect through Dental Awareness (PANDA) is a coalition founded in 2001 by dental professionals. Its goal is to create an atmosphere of understanding in dentistry and other professions that will result in reducing neglect and abuse through early identification of victims and prompt and appropriate interventions. The program was initiated by the Maryland State Dental Association and was adopted by the American Dental Association. Training programs for dental professionals include a 2-hour presentation that uses case studies and discussion to provide orientation to the identification of neglect, child abuse, partner abuse, and vulnerable adult abuse. More information is available at www.ada.org.[7]

Give Back a Smile

Give Back a Smile is a program of the American Academy of Cosmetic Dentistry. Members volunteer to provide restorative and cosmetic dentistry in the smile zone of the mouth at no cost to victims of FV who have experienced broken or lost teeth through violence. Volunteer dental laboratory technicians provide needed prosthetic appliances in cooperation with the volunteer dentist. The program began in 2006, and between 2006 and 2009 it has provided $4 million in free dental care. This service is especially helpful in removing the constant reminder of FV; bruises heal, but broken teeth can remain for a lifetime. More information is available at www.aacd.com.

Agencies/Associations for Consultation and Referral Related to Documentation

The following organizations may be available for consultation or referral regarding identification, documentation, and testimony related to the outcomes of FV:

- The American Board of Forensic Odontology (www.abfo.org) establishes standards and certifies those volunteer applicants who comply with the requirements of the board. Their purpose is to identify forensic scientists who are qualified to provide services for the judicial and executive branches of government. The board provides referral, at no cost, to attorneys seeking scientific expert witnesses.
- The American Society of Forensic Odontology (www.asfo.org), one of the largest organizations of its type, is open to worldwide membership. It provides continuing education on topics such as the role of dentists in bite-mark documentation.
- The American Association of Forensic Science (www.aafs.org) includes a section for odontologists and provides an opportunity for dentists to interact with other health professionals working in the area of forensics.

CONCLUSIONS

Because a high percentage of injuries sustained in FV involve the head and neck, dentists and members of the dental team can be invaluable allies in the detection and documentation of FV, and they are the only health professionals who can restore broken teeth that can be a constant reminder of the violence. Including dentists in a team of health professionals addressing issues of FV will add important dimensions of documentation, identification, and intervention.

REFERENCES

1. Behavioral Risk Factor Surveillance System Web site. http://apps.nccd.cdc.gov/BRFSS. Accessed March 14, 2010.
2. Le BT, Dierks EJ, Ueek LD, Potter H, Potter BF. Maxillofacial injuries associated with domestic violence. *J Oral Maxillofac Surg.* 1996;59:1227.
3. Tjaden P, Thoennes N. *Prevalence, Incidence, and Consequences of Violence Against Women: Findings from the National Violence Against Women Survey.* Washington, DC: National Institute of Justice, Centers for Disease Control and Prevention; 1998:6–9.
4. Berrios DC, Grady D. Domestic violence: risk factors and outcomes. *West J Med.* 1991;155:133–135.
5. Ochs HA, Neuenschwander MC, Dodson TB. Are head, neck and facial injuries markers of domestic violence? *JADA.* 1996;127:757–761.
6. Nelms AP, Gutmann ME, Solomon ES, DeWald JP, Campbell PR. What victims of domestic violence need from the dental profession. *J Dent Educ.* 2009;73(4):490–498.
7. American Dental Association Web site. http://www.ada.org/prof/prac/law/code/ada_code.pdf. Accessed March 14, 2010.
8. American Dental Education Association. ADEA policy statements. *J Dent Educ.* 2008;72(7):822.
9. Love C, Gerbert B, Caspers N, Bronstone A, Perry D, Bird W. Dentists' attitudes and behaviors regarding domestic violence. *J Am Dent Assoc.* 2001;132:85–93.
10. Stalker CA, Carruthers RBD, Teram E, Schachter C. Providing dental care to survivors of childhood sexual abuse: treatment considerations for the practitioner. *JADA.* 2005;136(9):1277–1281.
11. McDowell JD, Kassebaum D, Stromboe S. Recognizing and reporting victims of domestic violence. *JADA.* 1992;123:44–50.
12. Domestic violence facts. National Coalition Against Domestic Violence Web site. http://www.ncadv.org. Accessed March 23, 2010.
13. Halpern LR, Dodson TB. A predictive model to identify women with injuries related to intimate partner violence. *JADA.* 2006;137:604–609.
14. Isaac NE, Enos VP. Documenting domestic violence: how health care providers can help victims. National Institute of Justice, US Department of Justice;

September 2001. Available at http://www1.cj.msu.edu/~outreach/mvaa/Domestic%20Violence/Related%20Articles/Documenting%20Domestic%20Violence.pdf. Accessed October 11, 2010.

15. Senn DR, McDowell JD, Alder ME. Dentistry's role in the recognition and reporting of domestic violence, abuse, neglect. *Dent Clin North Am Forensic Odontol.* 2001;45(2):343–363, ix.

16. Fenton SJ, Bouquot JE, Unkel JH. Orofacial considerations for pediatric, adult, and elderly victims of abuse. *Emerg Med Clin North Am.* 2000;18(3):601–617.

17. Kenney JP. Domestic violence: a complex health care issue for dentistry today. *Forensic Sci Int.* 2006;159(1):S121–S125.

18. Wiseman M. The role of the dentist in recognizing elder abuse. *JADC.* 2008; 74(8):715–720.

19. Sweet DJ. Bitemark evidence. In: *Manual of Forensic Odontology.* 3rd ed. 1997.

20. Dailey JC, Bowers CM. Aging of bitemarks: a literature review. In: *Manual of Forensic Odontology.* 3rd ed. 1997.

21. Dougall A, Fiske J. Surviving child sexual abuse: the relevance to dental practice. *Dent Update.* 2009;36:294–304.

Chapter 20

Dealing with Perpetrators

Peter Cronholm, MD, MSCE
Tony Lapp, LCSW
Lois S. Cronholm, PhD

INTRODUCTION

Intimate partner violence (IPV) is a complex entity. The common response to it has been based largely on the role of males as perpetrators and females as victims. This response has been validated both by publicity and by the data that show in violence-related deaths from suicides, homicides, and armed conflicts that women are predominantly the victims. The National Family Violence Survey and surveys by the Centers for Disease Control and Prevention (CDC) suggest that men and women report similar rates of IPV.[1,2] However, national data indicate that most of the injuries resulting from violence involve male violence against women and that this violence tends to be chronic.[3,4] In 95% of episodes of IPV leading to criminal investigation and 59% of spouse murders, women were the victims.[5] We do not know how often, in the case of spouse murders in which the woman murders the man, that it was done as an act of self-defense.

Clinicians must consider the complexities of IPV from the perspective that defining it as a phenomenon of male perpetration and female victimization leaves providers and patients isolated from the realities of same-sex IPV, male victimization by female perpetration, and mutually aggressive relationships (although both of the latter are less common). The common and useful conceptual framework of IPV perpetration is rooted in explaining the dynamics of power and control in intimate relationships (Chapter 2).

Studies have indicated that both genders may be perpetrators and/or victims and the typology of male perpetration is complex.[6] For example, some male perpetrators exert control over all aspects of their partners' lives; others attempt to control only specific situations.[7]

For effective responses to IPV, health providers should include male perpetration in IPV as an issue that may have significant clinical impact on diagnostic and treatment modalities. Concentration on males as the predominant perpetrators is appropriate because the data support this role. Clinical interventions addressing the primary prevention of IPV focus on the high health-related impact of male perpetration against female victims, which is the most studied dynamic of IPV and the one for which we have the most resources. However, it should not be forgotten than in some situations, as noted above, females or same-sex partners can be the aggressors, whether the abuse is physical or otherwise.

DYNAMICS

In the 1990s, Michael Johnson developed a literature base for a conceptual model of IPV perpetration that includes the variability of violence manifestations.[6] His work has resulted in the characterization of two forms of IPV perpetration: intimate terrorism and situational couple violence. Intimate terrorism is characterized by perpetration behaviors that attempt to produce general control over one's partner. Situational couple violence best describes behaviors that are not part of a general pattern of control perpetrated against a partner but are more a manifestation of escalating conflict. Since most of the data on IPV perpetration is derived from convenience samples of perpetrators in the criminal justice system or from victims in IPV shelters, the prototypical image of IPV perpetration is most consistent with Johnson's description of intimate terrorism.

The proportion of total IPV represented by intimate terrorism is unknown. However, this dynamic is one that may lead to significant injury to the victim. Johnson[8] studied the relative proportion of his typologies based on different sampling structures. He found that intimate terrorism was least common in a general sample (11%) compared with court samples (68%) and shelter samples (79%).[8] Similarly, Graham-Kevan and Archer[9] found that 33% of a general sample could be categorized as intimate terrorism compared with 88% of a shelter sample. Another scenario is that of situational couple violence, where couples may be mutually aggressive towards each other. It should be noted that mutual aggression does not necessarily imply that the levels of aggression are equal, and subsequent risk assessment should examine differences in, for example, severity of assaultive behaviors.

DIAGNOSTIC CHARACTERISTICS

One result of the recognition of the multiple dimensions of IPV is the difficulty of settling on reliable IPV typologies with regard to the definition of IPV, diagnostic characteristics of perpetrators and victims, and the health effects of perpetration. There is no accepted diagnostic description of perpetrators and victims. Persons of virtually every race, economic status, religion, cultural group, and gender may engage in perpetration. The perpetrator in an intimate terrorism model is characterized as seeking to control the partner.[9] He may have low self-esteem and a sense of self that is integrally connected to his partner. Thus, he will often do anything to maintain control of the relationship. This is one reason that women are in more danger when they try to leave or break the ties with their perpetrator.

Males may present as either victim or perpetrator with injuries from violence or comorbidities, but these are not unique to IPV, and the relationship to perpetration may not be recognized unless the patient self-identifies or the screening process reveals perpetration.[10] Gerlock[11] reported that men in counseling for IPV perpetration used healthcare systems for multiple reasons, including musculoskeletal (50%), cardiovascular (14%), gastrointestinal (13%), nervous system (10%), dermatologic (10%), and pulmonary complaints (8%).[11] Close to a third of perpetrators analyzed believed that their symptoms of depression and anxiety resulted from their perpetration behaviors.[11]

Some males may be both perpetrators and victims, and it may be hard to distinguish between the two. One person may incorporate both victimization and perpetration, as when men remain affected as the victims of their own childhood abuse or as a result of witnessing parental abuse. Perpetrators are more likely to have been victims of childhood abuse than comparison cohorts.[12,13] In an analysis of 8629 participants in the Adverse Childhood Experiences Study conducted at Kaiser Permanente by Whitfield and colleagues, the risk of victimization and perpetration in people who had been victims of physical or sexual abuse as children was increased 3.5-fold for women and 3.8-fold for men.[14] Recognition of these patterns requires a shift in common perceptions and responses.

Sugg et al conducted one of the few studies that included identification of perpetration in the primary care setting.[15] She and her colleagues found that 10% of primary care providers reported never having identified an IPV victim, and 55% never identified an IPV perpetrator. Most primary care providers reported that they thought IPV was rare in their practice but reported higher rates when asked about the healthcare system in general. The study supports the well-recognized fact that IPV is more prevalent than reported or recognized and highlights the prevalence of denial among providers.

Many professional agencies support and encourage screening for IPV victimization based on the prevalence and the associated health-related comorbidities of IPV, as well as the recognition of the pivotal role of healthcare providers in identifying and referring victims for counseling. In contrast, the US Preventive Services Task Force (USPSTF) concluded that there was insufficient evidence for or against screening for IPV in women[16] (see Chapter 16). Neither direction nor support exists from professional organizations or clinical guidelines regarding screening for perpetration. Little attention has been directed to clinical efforts to address IPV perpetration. However, one might surmise that if the USPSTF considers screening for victimization as possibly not necessary, screening for perpetration would likely be considered totally unnecessary.

The healthcare provider must be aware that the screening discussed in this chapter may reveal that a patient is a perpetrator, a victim, or both, and that victimization also has potentially important health issues that may be masked by lack of knowledge of the cause. Just as specific methods are needed to identify perpetration, males also may be reluctant to attribute or reveal the relationship between health issues and victimization. More is known about the health-related characteristics of female victimization than of male perpetration or victimization, but it may be possible that some parallel processes exist in male victims. IPV victimization has a complex interaction with health, with an impact on physical, mental, emotional, social, and financial dimensions. Physical injuries may include contusions, lacerations, broken bones, and death.[11] Another long-term consequence of perpetration is transference of aggression to children who are then at subsequently higher risk for becoming perpetrators or victims of violence themselves.[17-22]

SCREENING

The primary care health provider may incorporate a discussion of IPV issues into screening protocols, but it is not known whether identification of perpetration will occur. A comprehensive screening program of males and females and of perpetrators and victims is a laudable goal of primary care practice. Complex screening issues are related to IPV perpetrators who do not self-identify. Although some health issues identified with male perpetration are recognized, they are not unique to perpetration.[11,17,23-26] It is hard to identify perpetrators based solely on health issues or personal characteristics. Most protocols prompt providers to screen new patients and encourage more frequent inquiry during at-risk times such as pregnancy (see Chapter 11 on IPV in pregnancy).

"Asking direct questions" is best done using funneling techniques, where questioning is structured from a broad, less threatening base to more focused questions that address specific behaviors. Clinicians may consider including IPV screening in the social history of both men and women. Our work suggests that it may be better to ask about victimization before perpetration.[27] This technique may make patients feel less threatened by the line of inquiry. All providers develop their own style for patient interviewing. We have found it helpful in training providers to have a familiarity with some scripted questions as they develop their own style of questioning. The data from screening women stress the importance of a nonjudgmental style of inquiry. Below are examples of questions used in the RADAR (Routinely screen, Ask direct questions, Document your findings, Assess patient safety, Respond, Review Options, and Refer) for Men instrument developed by the Institute for Safe Families:[27-29]

- "How would you characterize your relationship with your partner?"
- "All people argue. How do you and your partner handle disagreements or fights?"
- "Do your fights ever become physical?"
- "Are you in a relationship in which you are being hurt or threatened?"
- "Have you ever used any kind of physical force against your partner?"
- "Has your partner ever pushed, grabbed, slapped, choked, or hit you?"
- "Have you ever done that to her/him?"
- "Has your partner ever forced you to have sex or perform sexual acts which you did not want to do?"
- "Have you done that to her/him?"
- "Does your partner put you down or make you feel bad about yourself?"
- "Do you do that to her/him?"
- "Are you afraid of your partner?" "Is he/she afraid of you?"
- "Has your partner stopped you from going places or seeing people?"
- "Have you done that to her/him?"
- "Who controls financial decisions in your relationship?"
- "Do you share decisions over financial matters?"
- "Has your partner threatened to call immigration and have you deported?"
- "Have you done that to her/him?"

WHAT TO DO IF HE SAYS NO

For most patients this may be the first time a provider has asked about perpetration. We suggest ending a screening process that has not identified current IPV exposures by opening the door to future disclosures with a statement about our understanding of how IPV exposures affect people's health and that if the issue ever does arise in the patient's experience she or he can always talk to us about what is happening and we can try to help. Questioning about IPV perpetration has the potential for making patients defensive if not conducted appropriately. Patients may deny IPV perpetration (and most do) if they are not engaging in the described behaviors, do not recognize their behaviors as those described by the screening questions, are minimizing their behaviors, or are not comfortable affirming their behaviors at that time or in that setting.

WORKING WITH SELF-IDENTIFIED PERPETRATORS OF IPV

In cases where a patient discloses IPV perpetration, it is helpful for the healthcare provider to be nonjudgmental in his/her response in a way that supports disclosure and does not cut off the opportunity for further discussion, but that also does not condone the reported behaviors. Referral to an expert in dealing with male perpetrators is indicated. Most therapists who work with perpetrators are associated with the court system. Clinicians should be aware of the resources in their area.

An assessment of safety and lethality is an important step in the assessment and management of IPV perpetration. Campbell's Danger Assessment contains items that have been significantly associated with the safety concerns of IPV victims.[30] These include increasing frequency or severity of violence, use or possession of weapons, substance abuse, threats of homicide or suicide, stalking, violent jealousy, or controlling behaviors.[30] Providers need to be clear about their role if there are concerns about imminent harm to the patient's partner. States vary in terms of mandatory reporting requirements regarding IPV. A few states have mandatory reporting of all known exposures to IPV, while others limit mandatory reporting to behaviors involving weapons, and many require mandatory reporting of harm to children or elders. It is essential that providers be aware of local laws regarding patients exposed to IPV.

A particularly challenging dynamic may be encountered when both the victim and the perpetrator are patients of the same provider or practice. The clinician often learns about the violence from the victim first and then needs to decide how to approach the perpetrator or ask him or her to change primary care providers. Ferris used a modified Delphi method to develop consensus guidelines for providers in addressing IPV when both partners were patients of the provider.[31] The needs of both patients should be addressed independently. Discussing abusive behaviors with either partner should not be discussed with the other partner. Independent safety assessments and safety planning should be conducted with the victim before talking to the perpetrator. Providers should be aware that their relationship with the partners, since patients may influence their own assessment of severity and referral options. Some of Ferris's other works are important in the domain of co-management of partners when IPV is present. Ferris provided data demonstrating that clinicians were more likely to discount reports of violence from a female victim if they had a relationship with the male perpetrator, which may be another reason for clinicians not to treat both partners.[32] Of additional concern was the increased propensity for providers to intervene in unsafe manners based on their relationship with the perpetrator. Providers were more likely to recommend couples counseling or to interview both patients together to address the issues of abuse in the relationship; both interventions are contraindicated in cases of IPV and may actually cause an escalation of the violence.[32] Clinicians should refer one member of the couple to another care provider.

We recommend referral to community-based services with expertise in treating IPV perpetrators. Such expertise may be identified through compliance with a statewide certification process, where it exists. In states without such certification procedures, providers may follow the recommendations of state-certified victim services programs in identifying local IPV perpetrator treatment programs.

In many states IPV perpetrator treatment programs require participants to permit the program to conduct confidential interviews of their intimate partners. Treatment outcomes for such programs include not simply measurements of the participants' level of cessation of abuse but the opportunity for intimate partners to gather information for their own decision-making processes (i.e., whether the patient demonstrates a desire to change, stay in the relationship, or leave). Providers should have ready access to hotline information at the local and national level as appropriate. Part of providing a therapeutic home for primary prevention includes the assessment and treatment of health issues related to the perpetration, addressing comorbidities such as alcoholism, drug abuse, depression, anxiety, and posttraumatic stress disorder.

REFERENCES

1. Straus MA, Gelles RJ. Societal change and change in family violence from 1975 to 1985 as revealed by two national surveys. *J Marriage Fam.* 1986;48(3):465–479.
2. Centers for Disease Control and Prevention. *Intimate partner violence among men and women—South Carolina: 1998. MMWR.* 2000;49:691–694.
3. Tjaden P, Thoennes N. *Full report of the prevalence, incidence, and consequences of violence against women: Findings from the National Violence Against Women Survey.*

Washington, DC: US Department of Justice, Office of Justice Programs, National Institute of Justice; November 2000. NCJ 183781.

4. Bachman R, Saltzman L. *Violence Against Women: Estimates from the Redesigned Survey*. National Institute of Justice, Bureau of Justice Statistics; August 1995.

5. Dawson JM, Langan, PA. *Murder in Families. Bureau of Justice Statistics Special Report*. Washington, DC: US Department of Justice; 1994. NCJ 143498.

6. Johnson MP. Patriarchal terrorism and common couple violence: two forms of violence against women. *J Marriage Fam.* 1995;57(2):283–294.

7. Johnson MP. Domestic violence: it's not about gender—or is it? *J Marriage Fam.* 2005;67:1126–1130.

8. Michael JA. Conflict and control: symmetry and asymmetry in domestic violence. In: Booth A, Crouter AC, Clements M, eds. *Couples in Conflict.* Mahwah, NJ: Erlbaum; 2001:95–104.

9. Graham-Kevan N, Archer J. Intimate terrorism and common couple violence: a test of Johnson's predictions in four British samples. *J Interpers Violence.* 2003; 18(11):1247–1270.

10. Cronholm PF. Intimate partner violence and men's health. *Prim Care Clin Office Pract.* 2006;33(1):199–209.

11. Gerlock AA. Health impact of domestic violence. *Issues Ment Health Nurs.* 1999; 20(4):373–385.

12. Hunter J, Figueredo A, Malamuth N, Becker J. Developmental pathways in youth sexual aggression and delinquency: risk factors and mediators. *J Fam Violence.* 2004;19(4):233–242.

13. Clarke J, Stein MD, Sobota M, Marisi M, Hanna L. Victims as victimizers: physical aggression by persons with a history of childhood abuse. *Arch Intern Med.* 1999;159(16):1920–1924.

14. Whitfield CL, Anda RF, Dube SR, Felitti VJ. Violent childhood experiences and the risk of intimate partner violence in adults: assessment in a large health maintenance organization. *J Interpers Violence.* 2003;18(2):166–185.

15. Sugg NK, Thompson RS, Thompson DC, Maiuro R, Rivara FP. Domestic violence and primary care. Attitudes, practices, and beliefs. *Arch Fam Med.* 1999;8(4): 301–306.

16. US Preventive Services Task Force. Screening for family and intimate partner violence: recommendation statement. *Ann Fam Med.* 2004;2(2):156–160.

17. Dinwiddie SH. Psychiatric disorders among wife batterers. *Compr Psychiatry.* 1992;33(6):411–416.

18. Coker AL, Smith PH, Bethea L, King MR, McKeown RE. Physical health consequences of physical and psychological intimate partner violence. *Arch Fam Med.* 2000;9(5):451–457.

19. Campbell JC, Lewandowski LA. Mental and physical health effects of intimate partner violence on women and children. *Psychiatr Clin North Am.* 1997;20(2): 353–374.

20. Bennett LW. Substance abuse and the domestic assault of women. *Soc Work.* 1995;40(6):760–771.

21. Bennett LW, Tolman RM, Rogalski CJ, Srinivasaraghavan J. Domestic abuse by male alcohol and drug addicts. *Violence Victims.* 1994;9(4):359–368.

22. Testa M. The role of substance use in male-to-female physical and sexual violence: a brief review and recommendations for future research. *J Interpers Violence.* 2004;19(12):1494–1505.

23. Oriel KA, Fleming MF. Screening men for partner violence in a primary care setting. A new strategy for detecting domestic violence. *J Fam Pract.* 1998;46(6): 493–498.

24. Bacaner N, Kinney TA, Biros M, Bochert S, Casuto N. The relationship among depressive and alcoholic symptoms and aggressive behavior in adult male emergency department patients. *Acad Emerg Med.* 2002;9(2):120–129.

25. Coker AL, Davis KE, Arias I, et al. Physical and mental health effects of intimate partner violence for men and women. *Am J Prevent Med.* 2002;23(4):260–268.

26. Coben JH, Friedman DI. Health care use by perpetrators of domestic violence. *J Emerg Med.* 2002;22(3):313–317.

27. Jaeger J, Spielman D, Cronholm PF, Applebaum S, Holmes W. Screening male primary care patients for intimate partner violence perpetration. *J Gen Intern Med.* 2008;23(8):1152–1156.

28. Institute for Safe Families Web site. http://www.instituteforsafefamilies.org.

29. Basile K, Hertz M, Back S. *Intimate Partner Violence and Sexual Violence Victimization Assessment Instruments for Use in Healthcare Settings: Version 1.* Atlanta, GA: Centers for Disease Control and Prevention, National Center for Injury Prevention and Control; 2007.

30. Campbell JC, Webster D, Koziol-McLain J, et al. Risk factors for femicide in abusive relationships: results from a multisite case control study. *Am J Public Health.* 2003;93(7):1089–1097.

31. Ferris LE, Norton PG, Dunn EV, Gort EH, Degani N. Guidelines for managing domestic abuse when male and female partners are patients of the same physician. The Delphi Panel and the Consulting Group. *JAMA.* 1997;278(10):851–857.

32. Ferris LE, Norton P, Dunn EV, Gort EH. Clinical factors affecting physicians' management decisions in cases of female partner abuse. *Fam Med.* 1999;31(6): 415–425.

Chapter 21

Legal Issues Related to Family Violence

Kerry Hyatt Blomquist, JD

INTRODUCTION

Family violence (FV) (including intimate partner violence [IPV] and child and elder abuse) has a very real and devastating effect on the parties involved and their families. However, we are just now beginning to realize the impact of this issue on the overall wellness of our society. Statistics clearly demonstrate that the prevalence of violence in these relationships costs society in more ways than we have been willing to recognize to date. Approximately 1.3 million women and 835,000 men are physically assaulted by an intimate partner annually in the United States.[1] It is estimated that crime costs Americans $450 billion a year; IPV in adults accounts for 15% of that total cost, which translates into $67 billion per year. A study conducted at the Rush Medical Center in Chicago found that the average charge for medical services provided to abused women, children, and older people was $1633 per person per year. This would amount to a national annual cost of $857.3 million.[2]

For healthcare providers, the statistics are staggering and undeniable. Thirty-seven percent of all women who seek care in hospital emergency departments for violence-related injuries are injured by a current or former spouse, boyfriend, or girlfriend.[3] The level of injury resulting from IPV is severe: of 218 women attending a metropolitan emergency department with injuries due to IPV, 28% required hospital admission, 13% required major medical treatment, and 40% had previously required medical care for abuse.[4]

And the injuries are not just physical: 56% of women who experience IPV are diagnosed with a psychiatric disorder, 29% of all women who attempt suicide are believed to be battered, 37% of battered women have symptoms of depression, 46% have symptoms of anxiety disorder, and 45% experience posttraumatic stress disorder (PTSD).[5]

Until the passage of the landmark Violence Against Women Act (VAWA) in 1994,[6] this issue had historically been shelved as a "family matter." Finally, with VAWA, new light has been shed on domestic violence (DV), and the consequences of our ignorance of it. Along with a newfound understanding of the impact that violence has on society as a whole comes the natural next question: How do we stop burying this issue and take it out of the shadows? Should there be mandatory reporting of incidents to underline the seriousness of the issue and to take the reporting discretion from the survivor? What should healthcare workers do in cases where such violence is suspected? This chapter highlights the legal issues that medical service providers need to be aware of when working with and for victims of FV. This chapter also discusses trends across the nation, best practices for healthcare providers, and recommendations made by advocates for survivors of violence.

MANDATORY REPORTING REQUIREMENTS: SUSPECTED INTIMATE PARTNER VIOLENCE

Because of the prevalence of IPV in the United States, it is certain that healthcare providers will be confronted personally with the issue. How they recognize and respond to it is not only of critical importance to the safety of the victim but to their professional work as providers. Independently recognizing the signs of abuse is crucial. In a recent study, 92% of women who were physically abused by their partners did not voluntarily discuss these incidents to their physicians; 57% did not discuss the incidents with anyone.[7] Additionally, in four different studies examining survivors of abuse, 70–81% reported that they would like their healthcare providers to ask them privately about IPV because they are not comfortable self-reporting.[8]

For clear public policy reasons, healthcare providers and emergency department physicians are mandated to report any and all injuries caused by firearms. But the compulsory reporting of IPV without the express and targeted consent of the adult victim is still neither widely recommended nor practiced by states.[9] In 1997, the American Medical Association (AMA) announced its official position on the issue of mandatory reporting.[10] The AMA opposed the practice as a conflict with the profession's ethical tenets regarding patients' rights and physicians' responsibilities: "The American Medical Association opposes the adoption of mandatory reporting laws for physicians treating competent adult victims of domestic violence if the required reports identify victims. Such laws violate basic tenets of medical ethics and are of unproven value." Other clear concerns about mandatory reporting exist, the most important of which is the basic safety of the victim.

The most dangerous time for any adult victim of IPV is when the abuser is first being held accountable, and this naturally initiates when the event is reported to law enforcement. To "out" any victim by reporting his or her danger without the person's consent or before sufficient safety planning is complete increases the lethality of the situation substantially, especially when it occurs before the victim is ready to undertake these actions.[11]

Advocates against violence recognize that only the victim in such a situation knows the safest time to leave an abusive relationship. Thus, best practices suggest that healthcare workers should always provide education, support, and resources for a victim, but, as the AMA recommends, they should shy away from reporting suspected IPV to law enforcement without the victim's full knowledge and consent. The key dynamic of IPV is control: the abuser's control over the victim (see Chapter 2). A mandate that healthcare workers must report suspected violence without the victim's consent effectively shifts control of that victim from the abuser to the system. If the goal is to eliminate violence and empower victims, then reporting violence without the consent of the victim would seem to only facilitate disempowerment. To facilitate the empowerment of victims, the system must allow them to regain control of their own lives and make decisions for themselves, including the decision to leave or to report their abuser.

In addition to the basic safety issues, a woman's health may be further jeopardized if the batterer denies her access to health care to avoid mandatory reporting requirements. If the batterer knows that any suspected abuse will be reported to law enforcement, he may forbid or severely limit medical care. The victim herself may avoid proper medical treatment, thereby risking her own health, if such treatment mandates her disclosure of the abuse. Finally, mandatory reporting poses an even more significant concern for immigrant victims of abuse, who might fear such reporting would lead to the immediate deportation of themselves or their loved ones.

Lastly, one of the main arguments cited in opposition to mandatory reporting requirements is that such an action violates the victim's autonomy and refuses to recognize her as a competent, rational decision maker.[12] Instead of focusing energies and resources into removing the many barriers to leaving, mandatory reporting requirements force the issue by usurping the victim's ability to make that choice. Long-term prognosis in these cases is not favorable; ideally, those who choose to leave have time to plan, have assembled resources on which to rely, and have completed sufficient safety planning.

Most states maintain toll-free telephone numbers for receiving reports of abuse or neglect. Reports may be made anonymously to most of these reporting numbers, but often states find it helpful to their investigations to know the identity of the reporter if emergency follow-up is necessary. All agencies must comply with both state and federal statutes that enforce the confidentiality of abuse and neglect records, the identity of the alleged victim, and the privileged communications based on the relationships of the parties. It is strongly recommended that healthcare providers familiarize themselves with local and state laws pertaining to the reporting of suspected abuse because trends in this arena are fluid. State Web sites offer critical information regarding the use and availability of mandatory arrest statutes, and several reliable independent Web sites are available that provide further information on screening, recognizing, and responding to suspected intimate partner abuse.[13]

BEST PRACTICES FOR PROVIDERS

If cases of suspected abuse are not automatically reported to law enforcement officials, what are the best practices for providers? Accurate screening and response to the identification of abuse is critical. For example, the greatest risk of IPV for women occurs during the reproductive years.[14] Research indicates that a pregnant woman has a 35.6% greater risk of being a victim of violence than a nonpregnant woman[15] (see Chapter 11). In response to this, the American College of Obstetrics and Gynecology recommends that all healthcare providers screen all patients for violence at regular intervals: during routine annual examinations, during preconception visits, once per trimester during pregnancy, and during postpartum examinations.[16]

Responsive training and screening is critical both to helping the victim and preventing violence, and, accordingly, screening needs to be seen as a priority for healthcare providers. Protocols for both screening and intervention should be developed, and all staff who come into contact with women, including social workers, physicians, public health nurses, or other health care or social service providers, should be trained in their use. Making the screening for and the response to IPV a priority is crucial.

MANDATORY REPORTING REQUIREMENTS: CHILDREN AND "ENDANGERED ADULTS"

Although IPV reporting requirements vary from state to state for the reasons outlined above, every state has laws that require people to report concerns of child abuse and neglect. Mandated reporting of IPV of an adult is a somewhat controversial topic, but most agree that a child is not capable of personally breaking the cycle of violence, and, thus, the intervention of law enforcement, state, or courts is necessary. A few states require all people to report suspected child abuse, but most states identify specific professionals as mandated reporters; these often include social workers, medical and mental health professionals, teachers, and child-care providers.[17]

The circumstances under which a mandatory report must be made also vary from state to state. Typically, a report must be made when the reporter, in his or her official capacity, suspects or has reason to believe that a child has been abused or neglected. Another standard frequently used is when the reporter has knowledge of or actually observes a child being subjected to any conditions that would reasonably result in harm.[18] In cases where a healthcare worker provides services to the entire family, this can be especially challenging. The mandatory reporting requirements remain inflexible, however, and healthcare workers must understand that their duty to the patient does not set aside their legal duty to report.

The reporting of elder or "endangered adult" abuse is also legally mandated in all states. Although defined differently depending on the jurisdiction, all healthcare providers and most individuals are charged with the responsibility of reporting the suspected abuse or neglect of those adults older than 18 years, who, for reasons of age, mental health ability, or infirmity, are considered "endangered" or high risk.[19] The clear legislative intent behind this is to prevent the abuse of a vulnerable group of individuals, who, not unlike child abuse victims, would be reluctant or unable to self-report. Most states have Adult protective services programs that run in conjunction with local and state courts and investigators who follow up on such reports, and they mandate the reporting of abuse in this vulnerable group.[20]

EMERGENCY LEGAL RELIEF: UNDERSTANDING THE OPTIONS AVAILABLE

What kind of emergency legal relief is available to victims when they decide to self-report? How can healthcare providers advise victims? Generally, "stay away orders" meant for personal safety can be categorized as either civil or criminal. When a criminal charge is investigated and filed, or an arrest is made, the court frequently imposes a "no contact order" on the defendant. This order precludes the defendant/abuser from making any contact at all with the victim in the case, as long as the criminal case is pending against the defendant. The purpose of this order is not only to preserve the safety of the victim, whose safety is at a higher risk once the abuse is reported, but also to keep the defendant from "tampering" with the state's evidence: the victim in a criminal case. This order is a part of the existing criminal case against the defendant, and, thus, its longevity reflects the status of the legal case; it is not initiated or perpetuated by the alleged victim.

Similar to a "no contact order" is a civil protection order. This is also a "stay away" order for personal safety, but it is initiated and perpetuated by the petitioner/victim. Although the legal specifics vary according to the state statutory language, each state provides this emergency remedy to the petitioner/victim, independent of any criminal action. Protection orders offer a comprehensive remedy for victims that can include both personal safety and the economic relief necessary to stay away from the abuser. This "holistic" approach has proven effective: reports indicate that 86% of the women who receive a protection order state the abuse either stopped or was greatly reduced.[21] Civil protection orders can be initiated without legal counsel, are free of charge, and present a real safety remedy for victims fleeing an abusive situation.

Typically, the petitioner/victim, with the assistance of an advocate, can petition the court pro se (without counsel) for an order mandating that the perpetrator/respondent cease all contact with the alleged victim pending a further order of the court. In most circumstances this order, if granted, will remain in effect until a full hearing before the court with all parties present. This kind of order, again, is civil in nature and not contingent on the filing of any criminal charges or report. Other forms of relief are available as part of a civil order for protection, including, but not limited to, emergency financial assistance, the possession of a residence, vehicle, or other necessary personal effects, and, in some cases, emergency custody of children in common. Of course, controlling statutes vary by state, and best practices suggest becoming familiar with the protective order laws of your state and/or the legal services available in your area.

Generally, healthcare providers should familiarize themselves with their state Coalition Against Domestic Violence or other local or state DV direct service providers for direct referral. The National Domestic Violence Hotline[22] (1-800-799-7233; http://www.ndvh.org) is accessible from all 50 states and provides translators in multiple languages. That number should always be available to healthcare providers and patients alike and posted for all personnel in a safe place. This hotline also can provide local resources, including direct referral to an advocate who cannot only help with emergency legal relief but can also provide the critical safety planning, shelter options, and emergency financial assistance that many victims need when they make the critical decision to self-report.

Regardless of individual state laws, a healthcare worker should never ignore a suspicion or knowledge of violence. A healthcare worker should act as an advocate and encourage a victim to seek help by providing the victim with resources that can help her break free from the cycle of violence and control. An educated, engaged, and understanding healthcare worker can provide personal support, especially for those victims who are not yet ready to leave a violent relationship. Victims who break free successfully are those who are wrapped in both support and services. Best practices indicate that a healthcare provider who is well versed in the dynamics of FV in its totality and has knowledge of resources available can make a significant impact on those she or he treats and, thus, on society as a whole.

REFERENCES

1. Tjaden P, Thoennes N. *Full Report of the Prevalence, Incidence, and Consequences of Intimate Partner Violence Against Women: Findings from the National Violence Against Women Survey* [NCJ 1837810]. US Department of Justice Web site. http://www.ojp .usdoj.gov/nij/pubs-sum/183781.htm.
2. Miller TR, Cohen MA, Wiersema B. *Victims Costs and Consequences: A New Look* [NCJ 1552820]. US Department of Justice Web site. http://www.ncjrs.gov/ txtfiles/victcost.txt; Meyer H. The billion dollar epidemic. *Am Med News.* 1992;35:7.
3. Rand MR. *Violence-Related Injuries Treated in Hospital Emergency Departments* [NCJ 156921]. US Department of Justice Web site. www.ojp. usdoj.gov/bjs/ pub/ascii/ vrithed.txt.
4. Berrios DC, Grady D. Domestic violence: risk factors and outcome. *Western J Med.* 1991;155:133–153.
5. Danielson KK, Moffitt TE, Caspi A, Silva PA. Comorbidity between abuse of an adult and DSM-III-R mental disorders: evidence from an epidemiological study. *Am J Psychiatry.* 1998;155:131–133; Stark E, Flitcraft A. Killing the beast within: woman battering and female suicidality. *Int J Health Sci.* 1995;25:43–64; Housekamp BM, Foy DW. The assessment of posttraumatic stress disorder in battered women. *J Interpers Violence.* 1991;6:367–375; Gelles RJ, Harrop JW. Violence, battering, and psychological distress among women. *J Interpers Violence.* 1989;4:400–420.
6. Reauthorized in 2000, 2005, and currently under reauthorization consideration.
7. Caralis PV, Musialowski R. Women's experiences with domestic violence and their attitudes and expectations regarding medical care of abuse victims. *S Med J.* 1997;90:1075–1080; McCauley J, Yurk, RA, Jenckes MW, Ford DE. Inside 'Pandora's box': abused women's experiences with clinicians and health services. *Arch Intern Med.* 1998;13:549–555; Friedman LS et al., Inquiry about victimization experiences: a survey of patient preferences and physician practices. *Arch Intern Med.* 1992;152; Rodriguez M et al. Breaking the silence: battered women's perspectives on medical care. *Arch Fam Med.* 1996;5:153.
8. Ibid.
9. Seven states (Florida, Hawaii, Missouri, Nebraska, North Carolina, Ohio, and Tennessee) mandate reporting by healthcare personnel of injuries that they have reason to believe are the consequence of an act of violence, with some stating the injury must be grave or the act must appear illegal before the requirement to report applies.

10. American Medical Association. American Medical Association diagnostic and treatment guidelines on domestic violence. *Arch Fam Med.* 1992;1:39–47.

11. Rodriguez M, Bauer H, McLoughlin E, Grumbach K. Screening and intervention for intimate partner abuse: practices and attitudes of primary care physicians. *JAMA.* 1999;282(5):468–474.

12. Iavicoli LG. Mandatory reporting of domestic violence: the law, friend or foe? *Mt Sinai J Med.* 2005;72:229–230.

13. American Academy of Orthopaedic Surgeons Web site. http://www.aaos.org/about/abuse/ststatut.asp; http://www.womenslaw.org; American Bar Association http://www.abanet.org/domviol/home.html as examples.

14. Gelles RJ. Violence and pregnancy: are pregnant women at greater risk of abuse? *J Marriage Fam.* 1998;50:841–847.

15. Ibid.

16. American College of Obstetricians and Gynecologists and Centers for Disease Control and Prevention Work Group on the Prevention of Violence During Pregnancy. Intimate partner violence during pregnancy: A guide for clinicians. Available at http://www.cdc.gov/reproductivehealth/violence/Intimate Partner Violence/index. htm. Accessed January 9, 2008.

17. For an update on current states' requirements, see the searchable database provided by the Child Welfare Information Gateway at www.childwelfare.gov. The Gateway is the successor to the National Clearinghouse on Child Abuse and Neglect Information and is administered by the US Department of Health and Human Services.

18. A great resource for finding an individual state's law on mandatory reporting of child abuse and neglect is www.childwelfare.gov. This Web site for the US Department of Health and Human Services includes a report that outlines and summarizes each state's law on reporting child abuse and neglect.

19. For instance, in Indiana, an "endangered adult" is an individual who is (1) at least 18 years of age, (2) unable by reason of a physical or mental incapacity of providing or directing the provision of self-care, and (3) harmed or threatened with harm as a result of neglect, battery, or exploitation of the individual's personal services or property. Ind. Code § 12-10-3-2.

20. For example, in Indiana, a person who believes or has reason to believe an endangered adult is the victim of battery, neglect, or exploitation but knowingly fails to report the facts supporting that belief to the appropriate social services or law enforcement entities commits a Class B misdemeanor. Ind. Code § 35-46-1-13.

21. Ptacek J. Battered women in the courtroom: the power of judicial response. Boston, MA: Northeastern University Press; 1999; Chesney-Lind M. *Ptacek,* Battered women in the courtroom: the power of judicial response [review]. *Crime Law Soc Change.* 2001;35:363.

22. National Domestic Violence Hotline Web site. http://www.ndvh.org.

Chapter 22

Global Aspects of Family Violence

Rose S. Fife, MD, MPH

INTRODUCTION

This chapter addresses sexual assault in the context of nonfamily violence as well as family violence because of the nature of the subject on the international scale. Family violence (FV)—child abuse, intimate partner violence (IPV), and elder abuse—and sexual assault occur throughout the world. Different cultural and environmental factors may alter the contextual nature of the abuse, but no country seems immune. In some countries, it may be more socially acceptable or more stigmatized than in others, but, for the most part, many aspects of FV are the same everywhere. However, there are two major contexts in which FV and sexual assault should be considered in different parts of the world: the "background" rates in a country in "normal" times and the effect of war and other tumult on the rates in "extraordinary" times. Coverage of the entire scope of international violence, especially as it relates to wars, military or civilian confrontations, and natural disasters, is far beyond the scope of this book. Indeed, these are topics that deserve and have received discussion in entire books.[1-6] The references just cited are by no means an exhaustive list. The goal of the present chapter is to provide an overview of the subject so that the reader can pursue various aspects of particular interest in depth on his/her own through the references provided.

FAMILY VIOLENCE/SEXUAL ASSAULT IN PEACETIME

As described elsewhere in this book (Chapters 4, 6, and 13), FV occurs at rates that, although representing wide ranges due to underreporting, are, unfortunately, fairly predictable in the United States from year to year, probably in large part due to underreporting. FV is described in all countries in which it has been examined. It is difficult to compare rates, given that the numbers themselves are so inaccurate even in the United States, but the impression is that a baseline level exists for each country. It may vary in scale from country to country, based on cultural factors and customs, changes in demographics, and economic climate, but, for the most part, these levels are probably fairly stable. The World Health Organization (WHO) conducted a remarkable, extensive, multinational study among 24,000 women at 15 sites in 10 countries: Bangladesh, Brazil, Ethiopia, Japan, Namibia, Peru, Samoa, Serbia and Montenegro, Thailand, and the United Republic of Tanzania.[7] According to the authors,

> The WHO Study was designed to address some of the major gaps in international research on violence against women. Specifically, the study aims were to: 1) estimate the prevalence of violence against women, with particular emphasis on physical, sexual and emotional violence by male intimate partners; 2) assess the extent to which intimate partner violence is associated with a range of health outcomes; 3) identify factors that may either protect or put women at risk of partner violence; and 4) document and compare the strategies and services that women use to deal with violence by an intimate partner.

The study was conducted via questionnaire by specially selected and trained female interviewers. Not surprisingly, as shown repeatedly in studies, the core of IPV was the need of the perpetrator to control the victim, and the variants of IPV included psychological, physical, sexual, and verbal abuse (see Chapters 2 and 6). IPV was associated with a woman's long-term health (Chapter 7) and intensified, increased, or occurred for the first time during pregnancy (Chapter 11), just as has been found in the United States. Again, as is true in the United States, most of the abused women in these diverse countries do not tell anyone about their abuse. The people in whom they most commonly confide are close friends, neighbors, and relatives. The WHO study concludes with 15 recommendations, from promoting gender equality to developing programs that target primary and secondary prevention of gender violence to providing more support to agencies that help abused women and children.

Another large multinational study, called WorldSAFE, was conducted among 12,000 women in Brazil, Chile, Egypt, India, and the Philippines.[8] Data were gathered via questionnaires, and the demographic features of the violence discovered as a result of the study were disseminated. Again, overall findings were broadly similar to those of the United States.

In a study of 13,457 residents of 15 countries in Europe conducted via face-to-face interviews, the acceptability of violence against women varied a great deal among the countries, with a persistence of the attitude of blaming women for their victimization.[9] Rates of IPV in Europe have been estimated as between 20% and 50%.[10]

In Guatemala, IPV was found to be associated with increased adverse health outcomes later in life.[11] In Mongolia, IPV was widespread and kept out of the public view as much as possible.[12] Associations with poverty and alcohol consumption by the perpetrators were noted. Dating violence and rape were described among male and female college students in Poland[13] using the revised Conflict Tactics Scale.[14]

Plummer and Njuguna[15] conducted an "exploratory, descriptive study" to examine cultural factors involved in child sexual assault in Kenya. They noted the use of children in commercial sex work and sex tourism, the myth that intercourse with a young female child could protect a man from acquiring HIV/AIDS, poverty, the large number of orphans, often homeless as a result of the death of family members because of HIV/AIDS and, more recently, as part of the aftermath of the 2007 national elections.

HIV/AIDS has been linked to FV and sexual abuse around the world. Women who are the victims of such abuse are much more likely to be infected with HIV.[16-19] Cultural practices, such as those of adult men having sex with young girls in Kenya, increase the risk of HIV/AIDS.[15]

FAMILY VIOLENCE/SEXUAL ASSAULT DURING WAR AND OTHER DISASTERS

Rape and sexual assault have been part of wars throughout history. They were described in ancient Greece and Rome, in China, during the Crusades, among Anglo-Saxons, in South America, Southeast Asia, Papua, New Guinea, Africa, and so on.[21,22] The rape of Lucretia during a lull in one of Rome's wars was an often repeated subject of multiple superb artists centuries later, including Titian, Tintoretto, and Poussin, as well as by Shakespeare.[20] Rape in the Trojan War was described by Homer.[21] Rape and sexual assault have occurred in multiple conflicts in the modern world. The rape and sexual abuse of Asian women by the Japanese in World War II has been described.[3] The Russians committed rape in occupied Berlin in 1945.[21] Rape and sexual assault occurred during fighting in Rwanda[4,21] and Darfur.[23] Rape was a major component of the so-called ethnic cleansing and genocide in Rwanda and Bosnia-Herzegovina and Croatia.[2,4,21]

Currently, gang rape is frequently reported in the Democratic Republic of the Congo. Numerous theories about the causes of rape in wartime have been proposed, including cultural associations, use of rape as a form of "strategy" in wartime, and humiliation,[21] but none has been accepted by a majority of scholars. As a corollary to wartime rape, rape occurs during other disasters or catastrophes, including civic unrest (such as the devastating postelection violence in Kenya in 2007 and 2008).[15]

SUMMARY

FV and sexual assault occur around the world, usually in type and character very similar to what we see in the United States. There are cultural and political factors that differentiate this brutality in various sites, but, for the most part, they are clearly similar in most ways. The types, severity, interpersonal settings, and outcomes are all too familiar. One might think that a truly substantive and multifaceted prevention strategy that worked in one place might work everywhere with appropriate modifications. Unfortunately, no one is close to devising such an intervention.

Rape and sexual assault have been part of war since time immemorial and are well documented in art, literature, and journalism, as well as in myth and folklore. Their causes remain unclear, but they undeniably are forms of aggression that humans have used during wartime. In some cases, rape might have been a part of the war strategy, but in many cases it was somehow a mass action that occurred as part of the tactics of individual fighters. One might consider wartime rape as a form of mass collateral damage, comparable to the explosion of a bomb that kills or maims noncombatants. The world in the present era is still a long way from ending this heinous crime, but human rights activists, scholars, politicians, and ordinary people must keep striving (and are doing so) to eliminate this vicious entrenched feature of war.

REFERENCES

1. Brownmiller S. *Against Our Will: Men, Women, and Rape.* New York: Ballantine Books; 1993.
2. Allen B. *Rape Warfare: The Hidden Genocide in Bosnia-Herzegovina and Croatia.* Minneapolis, MN: University of Minnesota Press; 1996.
3. Chang I. *The Rape of Nanking: The Forgotten Holocaust of World War II.* New York: Penguin; 1998.
4. Zawati HM, Mahmoud IM. *A Selected Socio-Legal Bibliography on Ethnic Cleansing, Wartime Rape and Genocide in the Former Yugoslavia and Rwanda.* Lewiston, NY: Edwin Mellen Press; 2004.
5. Block S. *Rape and Sexual Power in Early America.* Raleigh-Durham, NC: University of North Carolina Press; 2006.

6. Gottschall J. *The Rape of Troy: Evolution, Violence, and the World of Homer.* Cambridge, United Kingdom: Cambridge University Press; 2008.

7. World Health Organization (WHO) *Multi-Country Study on Women's Health and Domestic Violence Against Women: Summary Report of Initial Results on Prevalence, Health Outcomes and Women's Responses.* Geneva, Switzerland: World Health Organization; 2005.

8. Sadowski LS, Hunter WM, Bangdiwala SI, Muoz SR. The world studies of abuse in the family environment (WorldSAFE): a model of a multi-national study of family violence. *Injury Control Safety Promotion.* 2004;11:81–90.

9. Gracia E, Herrera J. Acceptability of domestic violence against women in the European Union: a multilevel analysis. *J Epidemiol Community Health.* 2006;60: 123–129.

10. Domestic violence against women and girls, 2006. UNICEF Innocenti Research Center Web site. http://www.unicef-irc.org/publications/pdf/digest6e.pdf. Accessed December 13, 2009.

11. Castro I, et al. Prevalence of abuse in fibromyalgia and other rheumatic disorders at a specialized clinic in rheumatic diseases in Guatemala City. *J Clin Rheum.* 2005;11:140–145.

12. Oyunbileg S, et al. Prevalence and risk factors of domestic violence among Mongolian women. *J Womens Health.* 2009;18:1873–1880.

13. Doroszewicz K, Forbes GB. Experiences with dating aggression and sexual coercion among Polish college students. *J Interpers Violence.* 2008; 23;58–73.

14. Straus MA, et al. The revised Conflict Tactics Scales (CTS2): development and preliminary psychometric data. *J Fam Issues.* 1996;17:283–316.

15. Plummer CA, Njuguna W. Cultural protective and risk factors: professional perspectives about child sexual abuse in Kenya. *Child Abuse Negl.* 2009;33:524–532.

16. Murray LK, et al. Violence and abuse among HIV-infected women and their children in Zambia: a qualitative study. *J Nerv Ment Dis.* 2006;194:610–615.

17. Dunkle KL, et al. Gender-based violence, relationship power, and risk of HIV infection in women attending antenatal clinics in South Africa. *Lancet.* 2004;363: 1415–1421.

18. Kim JC, et al. Understanding the impact of a microfinance-based intervention on women's empowerment and the reduction of IPV in South Africa. *Am J Public Health.* 2007;97:1794–1802.

19. Maman S, et al. HIV-positive women report more lifetime partner violence: findings from a voluntary counseling and testing clinic in Dar es Salaam, Tanzania. *Am J Public Health.* 2002;92:1331–1337.

20. Harris JC. Tarquin and Lucretia (Rape of Lucretia). *Arch Gen Psychol.* 2008;65: 250–251. Available at www.archgenpsychiatry.com. Accessed October 5, 2009.

21. Cohen MH, et al. Prevalence and predictors of posttraumatic stress disorder and depression in HIV-infected and at-risk Rwandan women. *J Womens Health.* 2009;18:1783–1791.

22. The PLoS Editors. Rape in war is common, devastating, and too often ignored. PLoS Med Web site. www.plosmedicine.org. Accessed December 1, 2009.

23. Chaikin J. Children of Darfur: a vulnerable population. *Int J Nurs Pract.* 2008;14:74–77.

Chapter 23

The Way Forward: National Needs

Betsy Whaley, MDiv
Ann M. Delaney, JD

INTRODUCTION

In the past 30 years, significant progress has been made in understanding the causes of intimate partner violence (IPV) and beginning the long journey toward eliminating it in our communities. Yet despite this progress, IPV (also known as domestic violence, or DV) continues to be a reality in the lives of far too many of our citizens. IPV service providers, law enforcement workers, child welfare agencies, the judiciary, and local, state, and national government officials all must ask the question, "What is the way forward?" In what direction does the United States need to go to address the causes of IPV, provide effective service and protection to the victims of IPV, and hold batterers accountable in a way that reduces recidivism? Additionally, because the various forms of family violence (FV) (i.e., IPV, child abuse, and elder abuse) described in this book represent an interrelated continuum, we must remember that we need to determine how to deal with the entire gamut of this public health nightmare.

At the heart of the efforts to eliminate IPV is the work of transformation. The presence of IPV in our homes and communities reflects the reality of "brokenness" at some fundamental level. This brokenness can only be ameliorated through the transformation of the systems that allow it to exist and be perpetuated. Seeing the way forward in the fight against IPV (and FV) requires that leaders and practitioners in each system strive to understand the issues of victims, offenders, and communities. In this chapter we look at some of the components of the work of transformation that seem especially important at this time.

COORDINATED COMMUNITY RESPONSE

The causes of IPV are systemic and include factors such as poverty, psychopathology, addiction, childhood exposure to IPV, and the deterioration of community, and the response to IPV is also systemic. The response system includes the criminal justice system, victim service providers, child welfare agencies, healthcare providers, local, state, and national governments, and the judiciary. It also includes community stakeholders, such as faith communities, educators, and neighborhood groups, to name a few. Although all of these groups desire a reduction of IPV and the improvement of our society, they approach the problem of IPV with disparate objectives and perspectives on how best to address the issues involved. The result is often tension and mistrust within the response system and a disjointed approach.

As a result of recommendations from the National Council of Juvenile and Family Court Judges in 1999[1] to implement the Duluth Model[2] of Coordinated Community Response (CCR), there has been a growing movement around the country to foster communication and collaboration among DV service organizations, child welfare systems, the criminal justice system, family courts, and community stakeholders to protect victims and hold batterers accountable. Rooted in the effort to implement CCR is the understanding that there is a relationship between IPV and other forms of FV. Although there is, as yet, insufficient research to evaluate the full impact of CCR efforts, it is clear that in communities where this model is being implemented there is marked increase in the level of communication and collaboration among the organizations involved.[3] Participants also report an increased understanding of the disparate interests and objectives of the agencies involved. Efforts like CCR seem vitally important as communities seek to build a collaborative and effective response to IPV. The kind of communication that can occur among agencies through CCR has the potential to bring to light gaps in the system that could compromise the safety of victims and their children, as well as to promote creative thinking and problem solving. Additionally, a CCR can help to identify the relationship between IPV and other types of FV.

COMMUNITY DEVELOPMENT

If we accept the premise that the presence of IPV and FV in our communities reflects a fundamental brokenness, then we must question the effectiveness of the current systems in fixing the problem. IPV continues to be a major social concern even after the expenditure of billions of dollars. Unfortunately, many of those dollars are spent in the delivery of services in a manner that turns the victim into a consumer and perpetuates the dynamic of maladaptive dependence. Although the movement against IPV was founded on feminist principles such as the empowerment of women, there is a danger that IPV (DV) service organizations (DVSOs) fall into the trap of institutionalization and lose their connection with the vital work of community transformation.

There is much to be gleaned from the model of Asset Based Community Development (ABCD) to aid our efforts to eliminate IPV. ABCD seeks to develop communities through focusing on the appreciation and mobilization of talents, skills, and assets that exist in the community. This model of development is firmly rooted within and driven by the community rather than by external agencies. Using this model allows a DVSO to promote sustainability and efficacy through mobilizing the assets of individuals and the community. Harbor Communities Overcoming Violence (HarborCOV) in the Chelsea community north of Boston is one example of a DVSO that has employed the principles of ABCD to the great benefit of victims and the community. At HarborCOV the emphasis is on individual and community transformation.

> Every day advocates see that a survivor taking control and responsibility for decisions in her life leads to powerful individual transformation. The crux of community transformation is increasing decision-making authority by the collective community, that is, those most affected by the decisions that are made. Communities benefit when local residents are effective leaders, and when more residents participate and become invested in decisions about which businesses operate in their community, how tax revenue is spent, how community problems such as domestic violence are addressed, and who best represents their priorities.[4]

At HarborCOV, victims of DV can transition into roles of leadership within the agency and the community, thus transforming their experience from one of victim to one of advocate. ABCD is fundamentally more sustainable than service delivery systems that rely heavily on large infusions of capital from external sources and points the way forward for DVSOs that are willing to invest in the work of transforming their organizations.

BREAKING THE CYCLE OF POVERTY

It has been well documented that women living in poverty are at much higher risk of becoming victims of IPV.[5] Although many DVSOs are good at connecting victims to resources to meet their immediate needs, it is a more daunting task to address the systemic issues that keep victims trapped in poverty. Financial literacy programs assist victims in gaining confidence in their understanding of personal finance. However, financial literacy without ongoing support and mentoring will rarely help a victim break the cycle of poverty. Around the country, DVSOs are working to develop and implement new models to help victims of IPV gain access to financial literacy skills and give them the support they need to negotiate the transition out of poverty successfully.[6] It seems clear that engaging victims and mobilizing community assets to ameliorate poverty, one family at a time, is an important component of the effort to end the generational cycle of violence for children.

One promising approach to helping victims break the cycle of violence by promoting financial independence involves adapting a model that is being used in communities in the United States, Canada, and Australia to help end the cycle of poverty. These "Bridges Communities"[7] are working to educate their residents about the causes of poverty and the barriers to overcoming poverty through the use of the "Bridges Out of Poverty"[8] and poverty simulations. The goal is to elicit the support of people who are financially stable and independent in supporting and encouraging individuals and families as they make the transition out of poverty. At the same time, these communities identify and train those living in poverty using the curriculum, "Getting Ahead in a Just Gettin' by World."[9] After participants complete the Getting Ahead training, they are matched with mentors who are trained to support and encourage them as they transition out of poverty. This "Circles of Support" model[10] holds great promise for use with victims of IPV because they are so often isolated and have no support system once they leave their abusive relationship. Although adaptation would be needed to take into account the dynamics of IPV, the "Bridges/Circles" model holds great promise for helping to break the intergenerational cycle of violence as children reap the benefit of their parent(s) becoming more financially stable and supported within a community. In addition, the community is given the opportunity to become educated about issues of poverty and the link to IPV. Because this model draws upon the strengths and resources of the community to help solve the problem of poverty, it has the advantage of sustainability.

MAKING THE CASE FROM A COST-BENEFIT PERSPECTIVE

The general public tends to see IPV as a personal and private issue and not to perceive the impact of the violence on the larger society. The Centers for Disease

Control and Prevention (CDC) has estimated that the annual costs of IPV to our society exceed $5.8 billion.[11] This number takes into account the cost of medical care, mental health care, lost productivity, and the loss of earnings for those killed as a result of IPV. This estimate does not take into account any costs associated with the criminal justice system. It also does not include any estimation of the "price" of workplace violence that can be directly related to IPV when an abuser pursues the victim to a public place and commits, or even tries to commit, an act of violence. When a person becomes a victim of IPV or FV, it affects not only that person but everyone within their circle of support. In 1993, the Department of Justice estimated that the cost of IPV for the criminal justice system was $67 billion annually.[12] Many DV organizations around the country face the tough economic reality that, in the face of shrinking revenues, governments and private funders must be educated regarding why it makes economic sense to fund DV programs. It is incumbent upon advocates in all arenas to educate themselves about the financial toll that DV takes on their communities. This knowledge is necessary if advocates are to be effective in making the case for why funding of prevention programs is in the public interest as well as in the interest of individual victims. Tools such as *Making the Case for Domestic Violence Prevention Through the Lens of Cost-Benefit*[13] offer much needed guidance for leaders who seek to build sustainability into their efforts to prevent and treat the effects of IPV.

In the same vein, those working within the criminal justice system must seek to increase prevention efforts while reducing costs. In 2001, the average cost for incarcerating a prisoner in a state prison system was $22,265.[14] The average expenditure per student enrolled in public education in 2005–2006 was $9154.[15] State governments are faced with the hard reality that dollars spent on imprisonment are not available for investment in programs like education and may, therefore, perpetuate societal conditions that contribute to DV. In the face of the high costs associated with imprisonment, many communities are turning to Batterer's Intervention Programs (BIPs) as an alternative to incarceration, with the hope of reducing recidivism. However, the effectiveness of such programs is, as yet, unclear.[16] More collaboration is needed between BIP providers and researchers to determine which models are most effective and which work best with different offenders. This kind of research is vital to assisting those in the criminal justice system to make appropriate and informed decisions about the most effective use of resources.

CONCLUSION

There is a tendency within systems to maintain the status quo, and, therefore, transformation requires a determined effort on the part of those involved in the work. It is a daunting task, but there is reason for optimism. Although the work of transformation requires a large output of energy, a tremendous amount of energy and enthusiasm are generated as participants in the effort begin to see the results of their labors. The work of transforming communities and ending IPV (and other forms of FV) will continue to move forward as long as those passionate about creating a society in which all people feel safe in their homes continue to ask the hard questions and build on the assets they find in themselves and in their organizations, governments, and communities.

REFERENCES

1. National Council of Juvenile and Family Court Judges. *Effective Intervention in Domestic Violence & Child Maltreatment Cases: Guidelines for Policy and Practice.* Reno, NV: National Council of Juvenile and Family Court Judges; 1999.
2. Coordinated Community Response 2006, The Advocates for Human Rights Web site. http://www.stopvaw.org/Coordinated_Community_Response.html. Accessed December 29, 2009.
3. Malik NM, Ward K, Janczewski C. Coordinated community response to domestic violence: the role of domestic violence service organizations. *J Interpers Violence.* 2008;23:933–955.
4. Holmes L, Davis J. *HarborCov: One Community's Effort to Build Comprehensive Solutions to Domestic Violence.* National Resource Center for Domestic Violence, Building Comprehensive Solutions to Domestic Violence, #19, 2006.
5. World Health Organization. *World Report on Violence and Health, Summary.* Geneva, Switzerland: World Health Organization; 2002.
6. VonDeLinde KC, Correia A. *Economic Education Programs for Battered Women: Lessons Learned from Two Settings.* National Resource Center for Domestic Violence, Building Comprehensive Solutions to Domestic Violence, #18, 2005.
7. *Best Practices in Bridges Communities.* aha! Process, Inc. Web site. http://www. ahaprocess.com/Community_Programs/Best_Practices/. Accessed February, 13, 2010.
8. Payne RK, DeVol P, Dreussi Smith T. *Bridges Out of Poverty: Strategies for Professionals and Communities.* Highlands, TX: aha! Process, Inc.; 2001.
9. Devol P. *Getting Ahead in a Just-Gettin'-By World: Building Your Resources for a Better Life.* Highlands, TX: aha! Process, Inc.; 2007.
10. *Circles Campaign.* Move The Mountain Leadership Center Web site. http://www. movethemountain.org/circlescampaign.aspx. Accessed February 22, 2010.
11. Department of Health and Human Services, Centers for Disease Control and Prevention, National Center for Injury Prevention and Control. *Costs of Intimate Partner Violence Against Women in the United States.* Atlanta, GA: US DHHS; 2003:32.
12. US Department of Justice, Office of Justice Programs, National Institute of Justice. *Victim Costs and Consequences: A New Look.* Washington, DC: US Department of Justice; 1993:19.

13. Transforming Communities Technical Assistance, Technical Resource Center. *Making the Case for Domestic Violence Prevention Through the Lens of Cost-Benefit.* San Rafael, CA: Transforming Communities Technical Assistance, Technical Resource Center; 2006.

14. US Department of Justice, Office of Justice Programs, Bureau of Justice Statistics, Special Report. *State Prison Expenditures, 2001.* Washington, DC: US Department of Justice; June 2004.

15. US Department of Education, National Center for Education Statistics. *Digest of Education Statistics, 2008* (NCES 2009-020), Chapter 2 and Table 179. Washington, DC: US Department of Education; 2008.

16. Eckhardt CI, Murphy C, Black D, Suhr L. Intervention programs for perpetrators of intimate partner violence: conclusions from a clinical research perspective. *Public Health Rep.* 2006;121(14):369–381.

Chapter 24

The Way Forward: International Needs

Rose S. Fife, MD, MPH

INTRODUCTION

As noted in Chapter 22, the World Health Organization (WHO) Multi-Country Study on Women's Health and Domestic Violence, published in 2005, is an outstanding international study of the status of domestic violence (DV) around the world.[1] The study was conducted in 15 different sites in 10 countries, including Bangladesh, Brazil, Ethiopia, Japan, Namibia, Peru, Samoa, Serbia and Montenegro, Thailand, and the United Republic of Tanzania. Data were obtained from more than 24,000 women by a cadre of trained local women at each site. The results emphasized the urgent need for action by a wide variety of stakeholders, including health workers on site, community leaders and governments, and international aid and philanthropic groups. The report indicated that "the wide variations in prevalence and patterns of violence from country to country and . . . from setting to setting within countries" show "that there is nothing 'natural' or inevitable about domestic violence." For instance, the proportion of women who report "ever" being physically abused by a partner ranges from 10% in the Philippines (1993) and 10% in Paraguay to 45% in Ethiopia and 69% in Managua, Nicaragua.[1] The authors added that "attitudes can and must change; the status of women can and must be improved; men and women can and must be convinced that partner violence is not an acceptable part of human relationships."[1]

RECOMMENDATIONS FOR CORRECTION OF THE PROBLEM

From the WHO Multi-Country study, seven categories of recommendations emerged, comprising 15 specific recommendations in all:

- Strengthening national commitment and action
  Recommendation 1: Promote gender equality and women's human rights
  Recommendation 2: Establish, implement, and monitor multisectoral action plans to address violence against women
  Recommendation 3: Enlist social, political, religious, and other leaders in speaking out against violence against women
  Recommendation 4: Enhance capacity and establish systems for data collection to monitor violence against women, and the attitudes and beliefs that perpetuate it
- Promoting primary prevention
  Recommendation 5: Develop, implement, and evaluate programs aimed at primary prevention of intimate partner violence and sexual violence
  Recommendation 6: Prioritize the prevention of child sexual abuse
  Recommendation 7: Integrate responses to violence against women in existing programs for the prevention of HIV and AIDS, and for the promotion of adolescent health
  Recommendation 8: Make physical environments safer for women
- Involving the education sector
  Recommendation 9: Make schools safe for girls
- Strengthening the health sector response
  Recommendation 10: Develop a comprehensive health sector response to the various impacts of violence against women
  Recommendation 11: Use reproductive health services as entry points for identifying and supporting women in abusive relationships, and for delivering referral or population services
- Supporting women living with violence
  Recommendation 12: Strengthening formal and informal support systems for women living with violence
- Sensitizing criminal justice systems
  Recommendation 13: Sensitize legal and justice systems to particular needs of women victims of violence

- Supporting research and collaboration
  Recommendation 14: Support research on the causes, consequences, and costs of violence against women and on effective prevention measures
  Recommendation 15: Increase support to programs to reduce and respond to violence against women[1]

WHERE DO WE GO FROM HERE?

Since the publication of the WHO Multi-Country study, the UN Secretary General's office has released a detailed study about all forms of violence against women in 2007, which included some primary prevention efforts. It also called on all countries to emphasize the need for reduction of violence against women and make what structural changes they could to accomplish this.[2] More recently, a document offering guidance on the primary prevention of IPV and sexual violence has been developed and will be released soon.[3]

Although differences among countries regarding violence against women are clear and may be the results of religion, cultural traditions, attitudes, and so on, numerous similarities are apparent. Issues of power and control, ego, roles, gender bias, and cultural norms include many familiar features from one country to another. The names of the religions, behaviors, and norms may be different, but the outcomes are painfully similar in the final analysis and condone the inequality of the genders. Primary prevention and other interventions developed for one region or group may be readily applicable to others, with perhaps only minor modifications in many cases.

REFERENCES

1. WHO Multi-Country Study on Women's Health and Domestic Violence. WHO Web site. http://www.who.int/gender/violence/who_multicountry_study/summary_report/en/index.html. Accessed April 23, 2010.
2. Expert meeting on primary prevention of IPV and sexual violence, 2007. WHO Web site. http://www.who.int/violence_injury_prevention/violence/activities/who_ipv_sv_prevention_meeting_report.pdf. Accessed April 23, 2010.
3. Harvey A, Garcia-Moreno C, Butchart A. Primary prevention of IPV and sexual violence. Background paper for WHO expert meeting, May 2–3, 2007. WHO Web site. http://www.who.int/violence_injury_prevention/publications/violence/IPV-SV.pdf. Accessed April 23, 2010.

Index